An Overview and Management of Multiple Chronic Conditions

Edited by Sevgi Akarsu

Published in London, United Kingdom

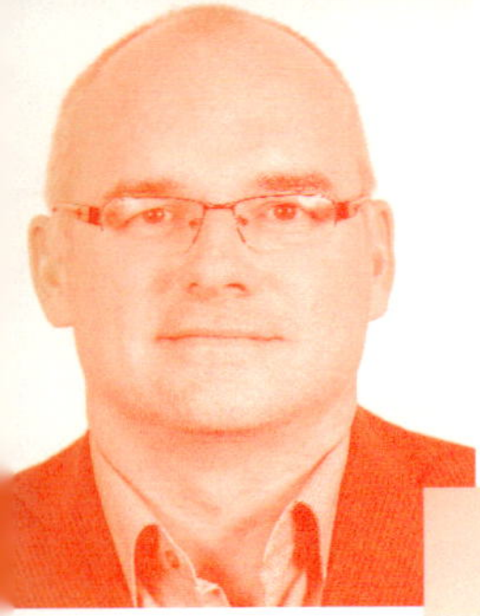
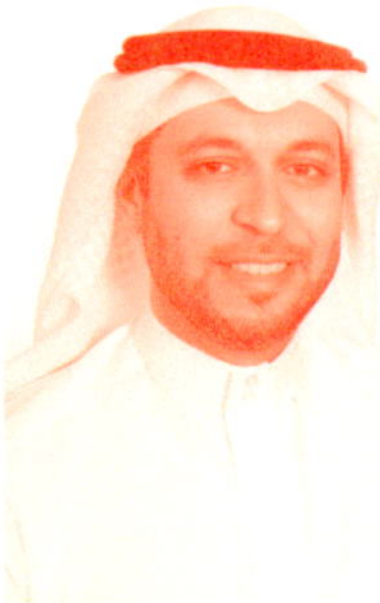
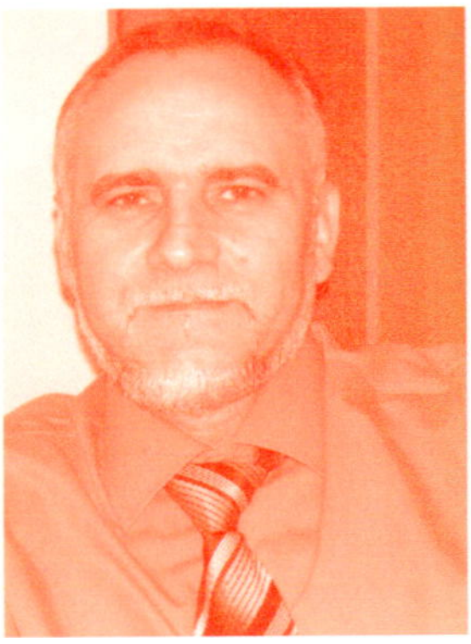
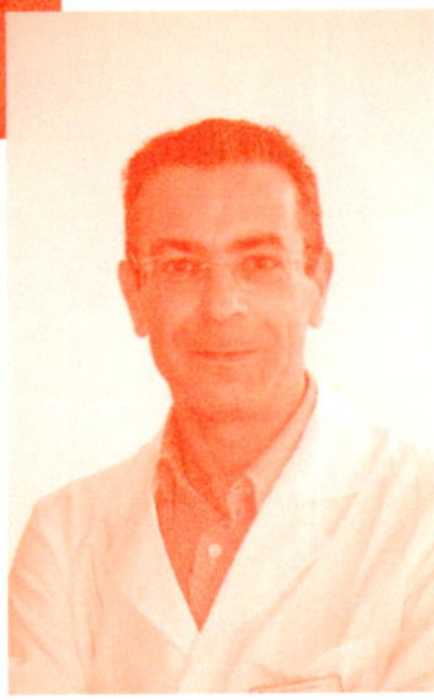
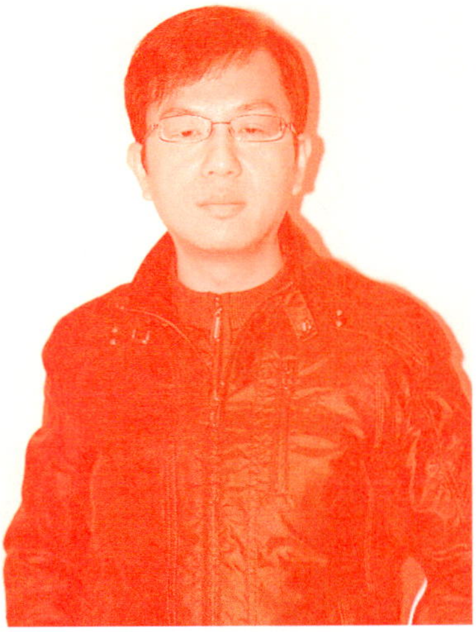
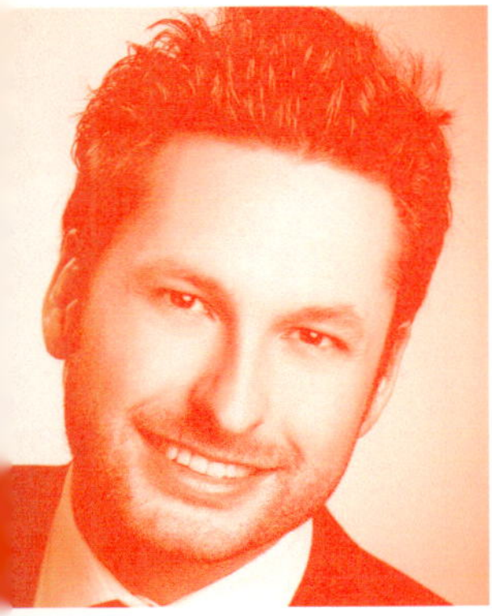
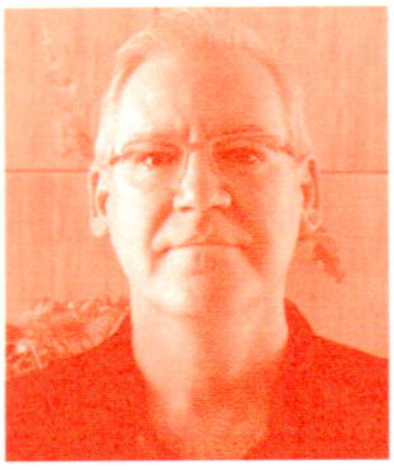

IntechOpen

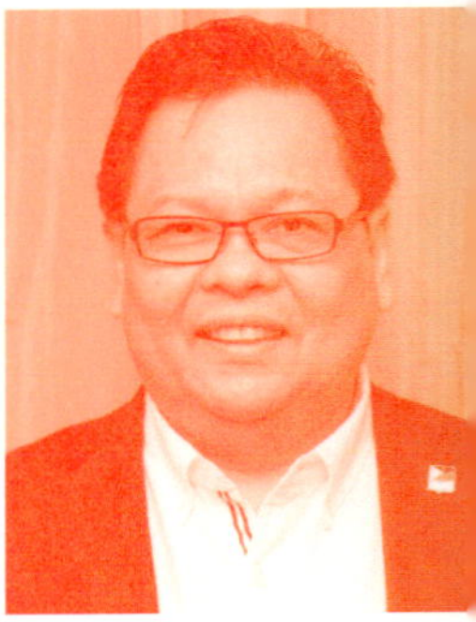
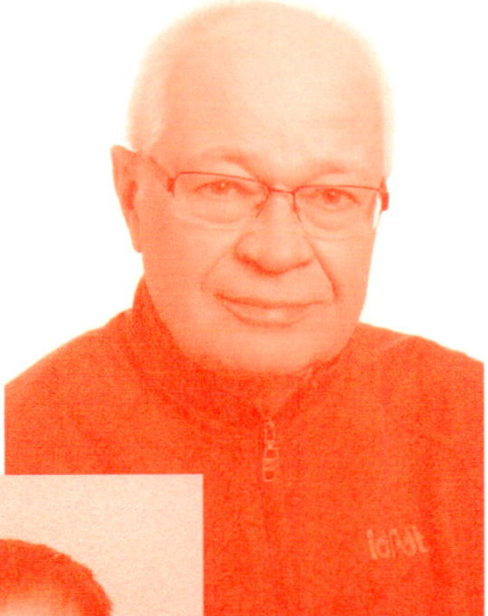
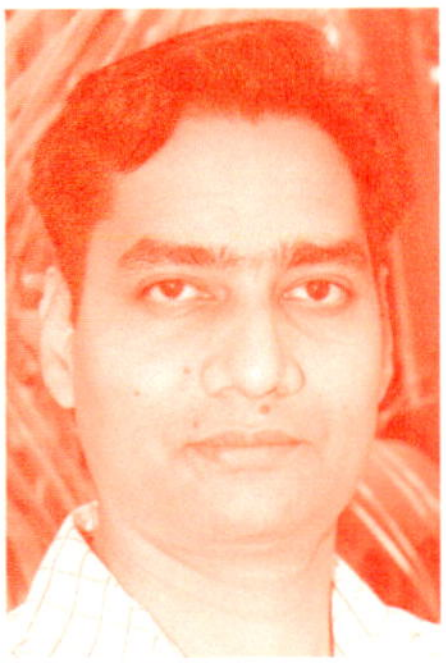
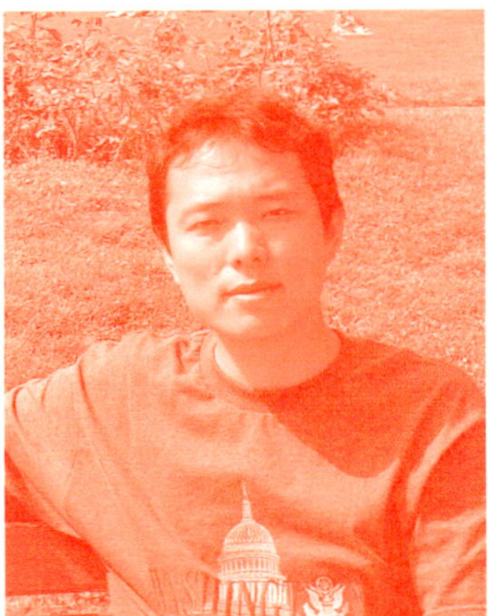
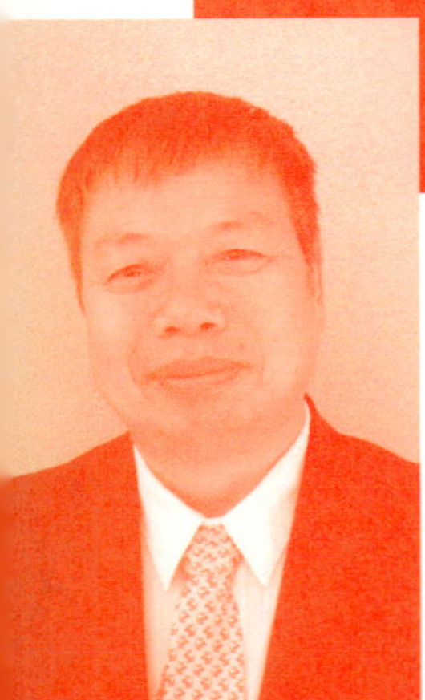
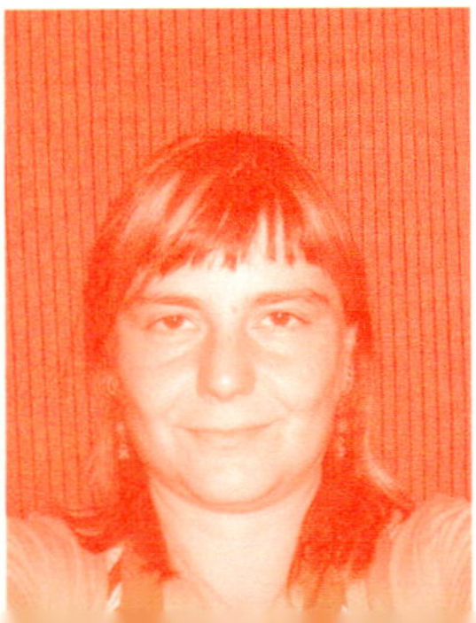

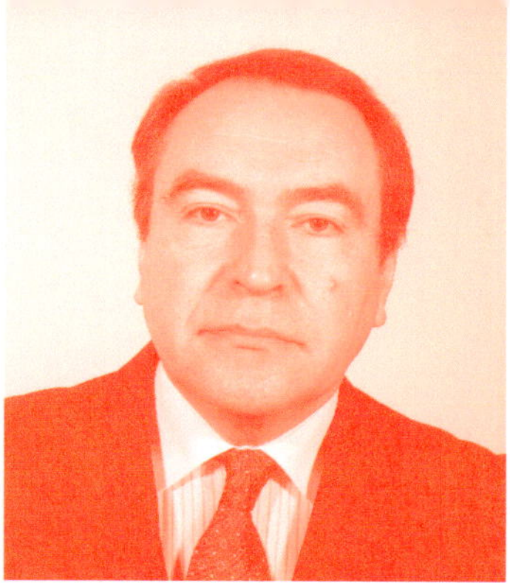
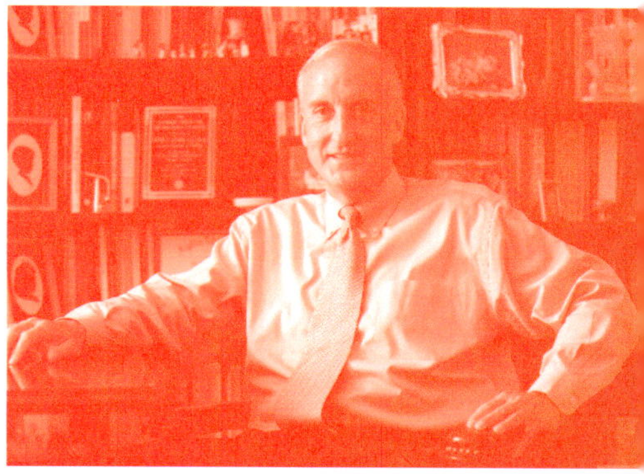
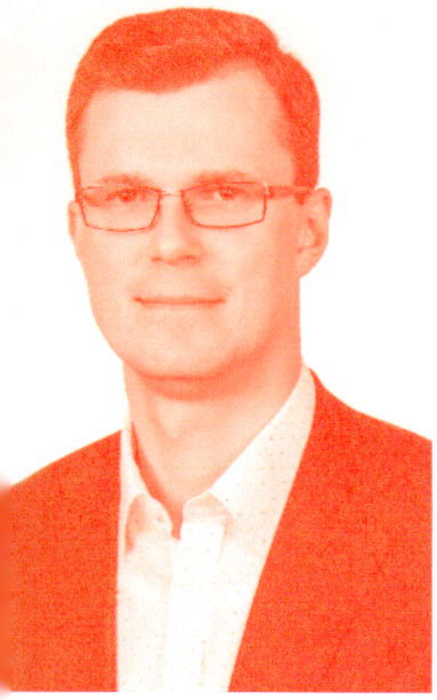
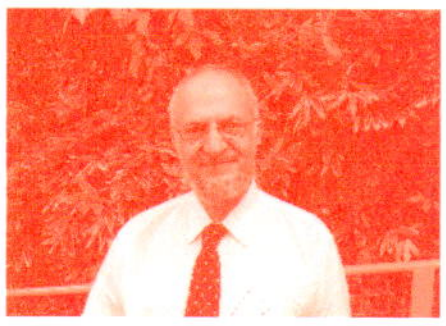
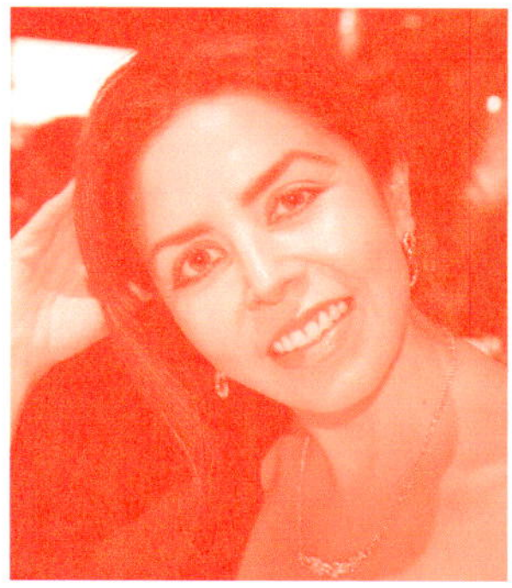

Supporting open minds since 2005

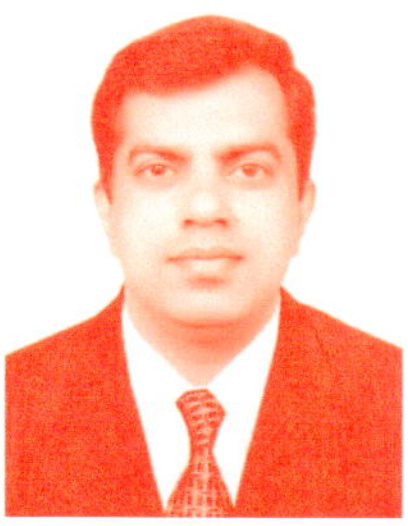
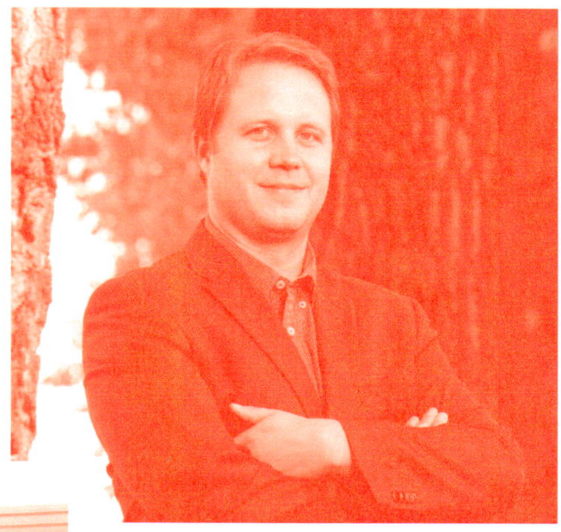
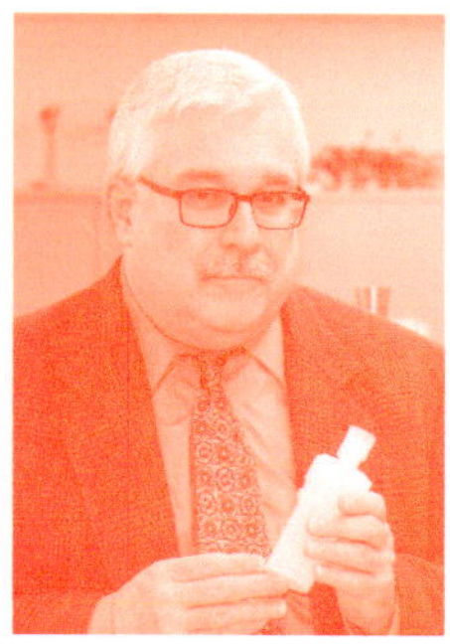
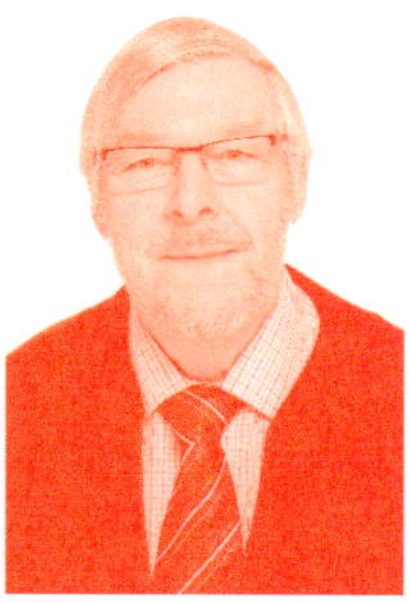
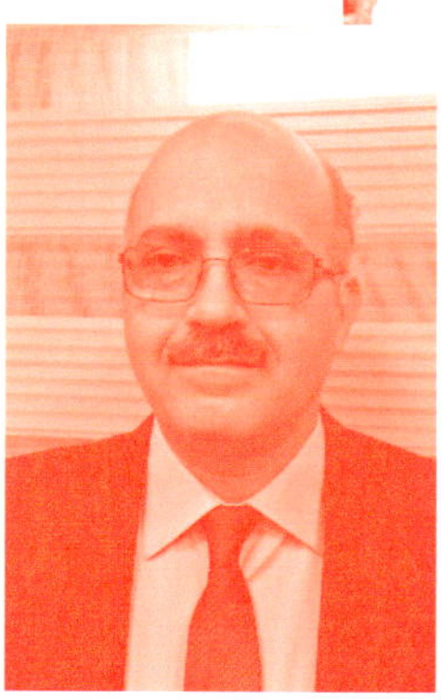
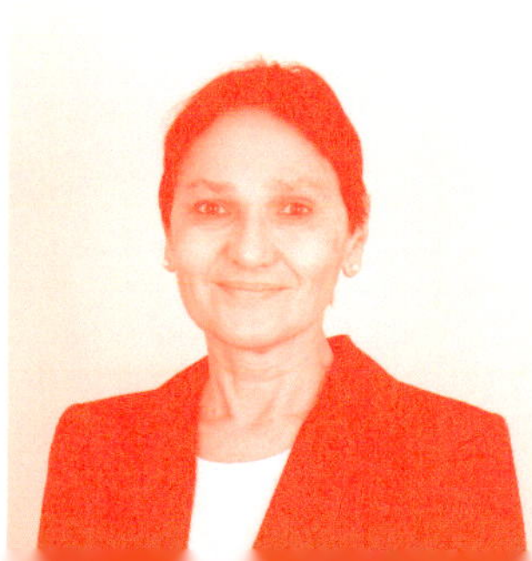
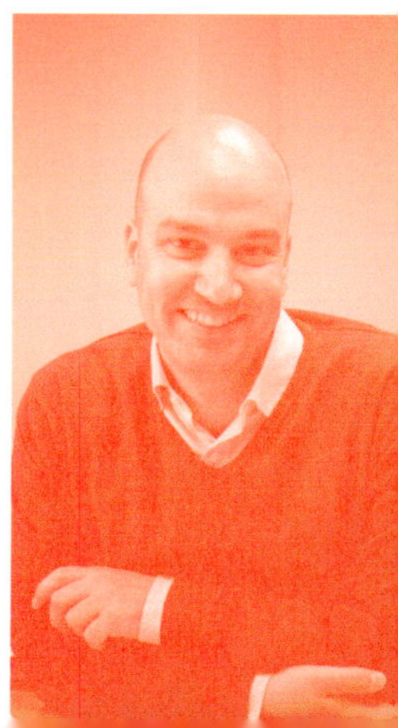

An Overview and Management of Multiple Chronic Conditions
http://dx.doi.org/10.5772/intechopen.83051
Edited by Sevgi Akarsu

Contributors
Daniela Simões, Raquel Lucas, Qingwei Ruan, Zhuowei Yu, Weibin Zhang, Emanuela Tudorache, Monica Marc, Daniel Traila, Diana Manolescu, Patricia J. McLaughlin, Chirag Patel, Ian S. Zagon, Gary A. Thomas, Sevgi Akarsu, Koh Iwasaki

First published in London, United Kingdom, 2020 by IntechOpen
IntechOpen is the global imprint of INTECHOPEN LIMITED, registered in England and Wales, registration number: 11086078, 5 Princes Gate Court, London, SW7 2QJ, United Kingdom
Printed in Croatia

British Library Cataloguing-in-Publication Data
A catalogue record for this book is available from the British Library

Additional hard and PDF copies can be obtained from orders@intechopen.com

An Overview and Management of Multiple Chronic Conditions
Edited by Sevgi Akarsu
p. cm.
Print ISBN 978-1-83962-310-3
Online ISBN 978-1-83962-311-0
eBook (PDF) ISBN 978-1-83962-312-7

For EU product safety concerns:
IN TECH d.o.o., Prolaz Marije Krucifikse Kozulić 3, 51000 Rijeka, Croatia, info@intechopen.com or visit our website at intechopen.com.

Meet the editor

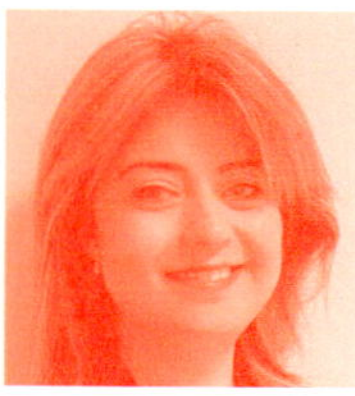

Professor Doctor Sevgi Akarsu was born on March 2, 1978 in Izmir, Turkey. In 2000, she graduated from Ege University Faculty of Medicine. From 2000 to 2004, she completed her specialization at the Department of Dermatology, Faculty of Medicine, Dokuz Eylul University, Izmir. Since then, she has continued her academic career at the same university. She has supervised several master's and postdoctoral students at the university, as well as published scientific research articles, case reports, and reviews in different journals including Web of Science Core Collection indexes. Her special interests are psoriasis, dermato-allergy, acne, urticaria, Behçet's disease, and photodermatology. Doctor Akarsu is still continuing her academic and scientific studies.

Contents

Preface

It is well known that the prevalence of chronic diseases is increasing rapidly worldwide, and approximately one-third of all adults globally suffer from more than one chronic condition. The prevalence rates of "multiple chronic conditions" (MCC), which indicates the presence of two or more chronic health conditions simultaneously in the same individual, are quite heterogeneous and show regional differences across the world. It is inevitable that MCC (also known as "multimorbidity") is becoming increasingly common as the world's population ages. As such, it is one of the greatest global health challenges associated with adverse individual, public, and financial outcomes, both now and in the future. *An Overview and Management of Multiple Chronic Conditions* is an up-to-date source of information for physicians, residents, and advanced medical students seeking a broader understanding of managing chronic disease clusters. The authors of the chapters come from many eminent centers around the world and are experts in their respective fields.

Considering MCC management in a broader context, the transition from a single disease-focused perspective to a patient-centered holistic approach may require considerable time and tremendous effort from health professionals and healthcare providers. Its burden to both the individual and society is increasing, probably due to lowered thresholds for diagnoses, advances in medical care, greater life expectancy, and possibly due to a true increase in the prevalence of some chronic diseases. Rheumatic and musculoskeletal diseases, which are among the most prevalent groups of non-communicable diseases, are highly variable medical conditions ranging from inflammatory rheumatic diseases and degenerative conditions to fragility conditions and regional pain syndromes. These diseases are the top three greatest contributors to years lived with disability in almost all world regions, as they are strong determinants of pain and disability limiting people's ability to manage their health. These diseases are also highly susceptible to MCC (especially in osteoporosis, osteoarthritis, and inflammatory arthritis) possibly due to their high incidence and low case fatality rate. They usually aggregate with a wide set of non-communicable diseases such as hypertension, cardiovascular diseases, dyslipidemia, diabetes, mental health problems, depression, and/or metabolic conditions. Recent studies also demonstrate that patients with chronic respiratory conditions, such as obstructive sleep apnea, chronic obstructive pulmonary disease, or idiopathic pulmonary fibrosis, commonly experience cognitive impairment as well. However, mild cognitive impairment is grossly underdiagnosed and undertreated by primary care physicians. Physicians who notice signs of memory loss, disorientation, gait impairment, or even poor adherence to pharmacologic/nonpharmacologic treatment should screen their patients for cognitive dysfunction and refer them to a neurologist for a thorough evaluation. Physicians should also be aware of prevention strategies for cognitive dysfunction in chronic respiratory diseases. In addition, special caution should be taken with cognitive-related comorbidities with which these respiratory conditions are associated such as cerebrovascular diseases, cardiovascular pathology, and diabetes mellitus.

Hearing impairment, hearing loss, or deafness is also one of the leading causes of years lived with a disability. Untreated hearing loss negatively affects communication and social engagement, leading to reduced quality of life. In addition, it is a potentially modifiable risk factor for dementia. Presbycusis, also called age-related hearing loss, is one of the most frequent hearing disorders among elderly people. Similarly, presbycusis-related tinnitus and cognitive impairment are common disorders in older adults that are almost always unnoticed at the early stage. Identification of the complex and mutual interactions among hearing loss, tinnitus, and cognitive impairment in connection with decreased peripheral hearing perception and central nervous system dysfunction suggested that comprehensive assessment, intervention, and treatment in consideration of these three diseases are important to decay aging. On the other hand, some cases of sensorineural hearing loss associated with many immune-mediated inflammatory diseases with variable prevalence in the population have also been reported. Psoriasis, one of these inflammatory diseases, is a common, lifelong multisystemic chronic disease that has multiple clinical types in a spectrum ranging from mild erythemato-squamous skin lesions to psoriatic arthritis. Like other diseases in this group, psoriatic disease is often accompanied by certain comorbidities such as metabolic syndrome, diabetes mellitus, cardiovascular disease, obesity, and psychiatric disturbances. However, physicians, especially dermatologists and rheumatologists, need to be more aware of the prevalence and clinical relevance of subclinical sensorineural hearing loss (as a neglected but important comorbidity) in psoriasis and psoriatic arthritis.

As a result of different physical, psychological, and cognitive challenges, multiple unnecessary or inappropriate drug use for self-care and disease management in patients with MCC leads to an increased risk of polypharmacy, inadequate treatment, adverse drug events, and drug–drug interactions. Recent reviews of multiple sclerosis show that the physical and psychiatric comorbidities (mostly hypertension, hyperlipidemia, chronic lung disease, depression, anxiety) are common and associated with disability progression, lesion accrual on magnetic resonance imaging, diminished quality of life, hospitalizations, and even mortality. However, little is known about how comorbidities influence multiple sclerosis-related treatment. Currently, there is no definitive treatment for this demyelinating disorder with an underlying neuroinflammatory disease process. It is suggested that relapsing-remitting multiple sclerosis is accompanied by decreases in serum endogenous enkephalins/endorphins and alterations in inflammatory cytokines. Low doses of naltrexone (an opioid receptor antagonist) to upregulate the body's own production of enkephalins has been shown by a number of clinical trials to be a safe adjuvant or primary treatment for relapsing-remitting multiple sclerosis. This alternative biotherapeutic continues to be associated with stabilizing multiple sclerosis, leading to improvement in peripheral spasticity and mental health composite scores without inducing any side effects. In addition, it does not appear to interfere with other disease-modifying therapies. Although traditional/complementary/alternative medicine practices have been often applied by physician/non-physician practitioners in recent years, it is highlighted that scientific investigations regarding potential benefits should be supported, and proven benefits need to be brought into modern medicine. There is evidence that traditional Chinese medicine for geriatric syndromes (including "Jia wei weng dan tang" and "ba wei di huang wan" treatments for dementia, "Yi-gan San" treatment for behavioral and psychological symptoms of dementia, "Banxia Houpo Tang" treatment for aspiration pneumonia, and "Da Jian Zhong Tang" treatment for chronic constipation) are partly accepted by modern medical doctors.

Every clinician, whether a general practitioner or a specialist who frequently encounters complex patients, should become increasingly aware of the clinical relevance and undeniable burden of multiple physical, cognitive, and/or mental chronic condition clusters. It is obvious that there is a growing need for population-based studies to determine the best management for MCC.

Dr. Sevgi Akarsu
Professor,
Department of Dermatology,
Faculty of Medicine,
Dokuz Eylül University,
Izmir, Turkey

Chapter 1

Introductory Chapter: Managing Multiple Chronic Conditions - A Patient-Centered Holistic Approach Rather than Single Disease-Focused Perspective

Sevgi Akarsu

1. Introduction

A chronic health condition is simply defined as a physical, mental or cognitive disorder that lasts more than one year, requires long-term monitoring and treatment, deteriorates quality of life and causes certain difficulties associated with the physical, cognitive and/or psychological disabilities. We know perfectly well that the prevalence of chronic diseases is increasing rapidly all over the world, especially in low-income countries. It is also a well-proven fact that three-fifths of human deaths worldwide are attributed to four major noncommunicable chronic conditions such as cardiovascular disease (e.g., heart attack, stroke), cancers, chronic lung diseases (e.g., asthma, chronic obstructive pulmonary disease) and diabetes mellitus [1]. Globally, about one-third of all adults suffer from more than one chronic condition. Although there is lack of a precise and consistent term and definition to describe such patients, "multimorbidity", "multiple chronic conditions" (MCC), and "polychronic disease" are the most widely used terms interchangeably [2–4]. Currently, "MCC" is still very popular, easily understood and the most commonly used term in both academic medical literature and non-academic environments worldwide [3].

2. Definitions and prevalence of MCC

The term "MCC" refers to the presence of two or more chronic conditions simultaneously in the same individual; however, the number of chronic conditions included in the definition and what constitutes a chronic condition varies greatly among studies in literature [4]. Some authors define MCC as coexisting conditions including diseases, symptoms and risk factors, while others interprete it only as the manifestation of end-organ damage (the endpoints of a disease) as a result of certain risk factors [5]. Therefore, the prevalence rates of MCC which generally range from 9.4–58% for the whole population (from 16–58% in UK studies, 26% in US studies, 20% of Australians and 9.4% in Urban South Asians), are highly heterogeneous and show regional differences across the world [3, 6–8]. In a large study of 25,293 participants from 14 countries (Austria, Germany, Sweden, Spain, Italy,

IntechOpen

France, Denmark, Switzerland, Belgium, Israel, Czech Republic, Luxembourg, Slovenia and Estonia), 50% of cases reported having MCC. Among these, it was observed that hypertension was the most common individual chronic condition (49%), followed by arthritis (34%) and high depressive symptoms (31%) [9].

According to more recently published National Health Survey Research report, 27.2% of US adults have multiple chronic diseases, with the highest prevalence in women, non-Hispanic white adults, adults aged 65 and over, and those living in rural areas [10]. Especially older age (up to 95% of the primary care population aged 65 years and older), low socioeconomic status and undesirable modifiable lifestyle factors (unhealthy diet, inadequate fruit and vegetable consumption, obesity, physical inactivity, household air pollution, sleeping other than 7–8 h, current smoking, alcohol use, etc.) have been substantially associated with the development of MCC [11, 12]. Similarly, in a large study using the National Health Insurance database and involving 333,294 patients, Wang et al. identified patients over 65 years of age, male gender, rural residence, low socioeconomic status, psychological disorders and high Charlson comorbidity indices as important risk factors for frequent use of outpatient services [13]. However, according to the data of respondents (n = 201,711) to the 2015 Behavioral Risk Factor Surveillance System, it was observed that more than 60% of adults with MCC were younger than 65 years. Compared with adults 65 years and older with MCC, these younger cases reported higher rates of smoking, obesity, asthma, cognitive impairment, depression, disability, poorer quality of life and poorer access to health care [14].

3. The impact of MCC on patients and health care systems

Both presently and in coming decades, MCC is one of the greatest global health challenges associated with adverse individual outcomes [2, 15]. Global Burden Disease Collaborators demonstrated that MCC contributing to the disease burden in high-income countries include ischemic heart disease, stroke, lung cancer, depression, diabetes, and back and neck pain. Similarly, these diseases are among the top conditions that contribute to mortality and morbidity in low-income and middle-income countries, but also communicable diseases such as diarrhea, HIV/AIDS and malaria play an important role [1]. It has been also well demonstrated that high blood pressure, high fasting glucose, smoking, high total cholesterol and high body mass index are the major global risk factors leading to chronic disease. Furthermore, certain chronic diseases occur more frequently in clusters, with associations of up to three-fold especially in developing countries, due to their high prevalance rates, common risk factors and/or a synergistic association between them (the most strongly associated clusters: Alzheimer's disease/depressive disorders coexisting with stroke, cardiovascular diseases and stroke alongside depression, and cardiovascular diseases/diabetes mellitus accompanying with long-term communicable conditions such as HIV/AIDS and tuberculosis, respectively). As can be understood from these chronic condition relationships, the coexistence of those may be associated with a common causal link, or they may be only weakly related or unrelated without a causal link between each other. It is generally thought that unrelated or poorly correlated diseases may occur together only because of their high prevalence rates throughout the world [3]. On the other hand, some authors mentioned that 'multimorbidity' is an integrated systems state reflecting a feedback of the person's genomic, proteomic, metabolomic, neuroendocrine, immune and bioenergetics networks to an underlying disturbance [16, 17].

Significantly reducing life expectancy with each additional chronic condition and affecting an individual's well-being, quality of life and normal functional skills, MCC may often lead to the appearance or worsening of depression and other emotional and cognitive disorders [4, 18–21]. Sheridan et al. mentioned that MCC groups including high depressive symptoms may be more disabling than MCC that involve only somatic conditions [9]. Ge et al. demonstrated that MCC associated with reduced self-rated health and health-related quality of life in all age groups whether they were young (21–44 years), middle-aged (45–64 years), or older adults (≥65 years) [22]. As a result of different physical, psychosocial, and spiritual challenges, multiple alternative, complementary, unnecessary or inappropriate drug use (multivitamins, multiminerals, nonvitamins or herbs, chiropractic/osteopathic manipulation, massage, movement therapies, mind–body therapies, special diets, and/or acupuncture) for self-care and disease management in patients with MCC lead to an increased risk of polypharmacy (simultaneous use of ≥5 medications), poor adherence to medications, cost-related nonadherence, adverse drug events, drug–drug interactions and inadequate treatment (underprescribing) [23–27]. Recently, Rahman et al. mentioned that many patients with MCC also demonstrated poor health literacy regarding medication [28]. Thus, in most patients, this complex relationship of multiple disorders is one of the main health problems and priorities worldwide due to a lack of joint guidelines, different screening and prevention requirements, a greater tendency to apply specialists compared to primary care physicians, as well as the increasing frequencies of emergency department presentations, hospitalisations, out of pocket healthcare costs and polypharmacy [3, 12, 29, 30].

4. Unmet needs, challenges and promising opportunities in managing MCC

Considering MCC in a broader context, due to the increasing proportion of older adults in the population, development of chronic diseases at younger ages and socioeconomic disparities in the distribution of MCC, serious challenges arise in terms of both the clinical management of patients and the organization of health systems [3, 14]. MCC is associated with a significantly greater increase in healthcare costs and resource utilization, doubling with every additional chronic medical condition [12, 31]. It will lead to the gradually increasing health, economic and patient burdens in particular low-income and lower middle-income countries expectedly although most studies and reports until now are from developed countries [3].

MCC is a special situation frequently encountered by global healthcare professionals, especially internists/primary care physicians, neurologists, respiratory/pulmonologists, pain specialists or oncologists, who spend more than three-quarters of their time in the treatment of chronic diseases and direct patient care. As the burden of MCC increases, the risks of unhealthy quality of life, poor physical function, healthcare costs and premature death also increase [32, 33]. Nevertheless, current traditional health systems and basic disease programs, as well as some of the most widely used health repositories (such as the World Health Organization and Global Burden of Disease databases) often adopt a single disease framework and rarely deal with co-occurring chronic diseases as a whole. Thus, the need for multidisciplinary approaches in the management of multiple chronic medical problems, rather than focusing on individual diseases, should be borne in mind by global healthcare professionals, public health professionals, healthcare providers, health policymakers and pharmaceutical industries [34]. Unfortunately, despite efforts in this approach, difficulties have been encountered due to the lack of basic knowledge of the etiology, epidemiology and risk factors of MCC and the variable effectiveness and cost effectiveness of different interventions [2, 4].

Despite the above-mentioned challenges, many comprehensive improvements and innovations (e.g., public awareness campaigns by using multiple channels and with participating well-prepared general practitioners; predicting groups at risk of MCC; development of health systems care guidelines, community based and integrated chronic condition care practices; caring the "complex chronic patient" which is defined by a particular profile presentation of chronicity where socio-economic, cultural and environmental dimensions play an important role; interventions enhancing problem-focused and emotion-focused coping; the self-regulation strategies of selection, optimization, and compensation; team-based care supporting physician-patient-caregiver relationships by healthcare professionals; patient-centered smartphone telemonitoring applications; fixed-dose combination pills/polipill approaches, and health technology applications in low resource environments) have been recommended by health care delivery system and health professionals, in order to prevention and management of MCC [8, 35–45].

5. Summary and conclusion

As the world's population ages, MCC is becoming increasingly common around the world. Thus, every clinician, whether a general practitioner or a specialist, should become increasingly aware of the clinical relevance and undeniable burden (with higher risk of the inappropriate medication, excessive healthcare utilization, and paying high cost) of multiple physical, cognitive and/or mental chronic condition clusters. However, the transition from a single disease-focused perspective to a patient-centered holistic approach may require spending considerable time and tremendous effort for the health professionals and healthcare providers. It is obvious that there is a growing need for population based research in MCC. Considering current approaches and strategies for screening, care and treatment of MCC, more studies and guidelines are still needed to improve our understanding of MCC, to best address the specific chronic health conditions that constitute MCC, to anticipate and screening groups of people at risk of MCC, as well as to increase potential areas for successful intervention and innovation.

Author details

Sevgi Akarsu
Department of Dermatology, Faculty of Medicine, Dokuz Eylül University, Izmir, Turkey

*Address all correspondence to: sevgi.akarsu@deu.edu.tr

References

[1] GBD 2015 Mortality and Causes of Death Collaborators. Global, regional, and national life expectancy, all-cause mortality, and cause-specific mortality for 249 causes of death, 1980-2015: a systematic analysis for the Global Burden of Disease Study 2015. Lancet. 2016;388:1459-1544. doi: 10.1016/S0140-6736(16)31012-1.

[2] Pearson-Stuttard J, Ezzati M, Gregg EW. Multimorbidity-a defining challenge for health systems. Lancet Public Health. 2019;4:e599-e600. doi:10.1016/S2468-2667(19)30222-1

[3] Hajat C, Stein E. The global burden of multiple chronic conditions: A narrative review. Prev Med Rep. 2018;12:284-293. doi:10.1016/j.pmedr.2018.10.008

[4] Navickas R, Petric VK, Feigl AB, Seychell M. Multimorbidity: What do we know? What should we do? J Comorb. 2016;6:4-11. doi: 10.15256/joc.2016.6.72.

[5] Willadsen TG, Bebe A, Køster-Rasmussen R, Jarbøl DE, Guassora AD, Waldorff FB, Reventlow S, Olivarius Nde F. The role of diseases, risk factors and symptoms in the definition of multimorbidity - a systematic review. Scand J Prim Health Care. 2016;34:112-21. doi: 10.3109/02813432.2016.1153242.

[6] Lim E, Gandhi K, Davis J, Chen JJ. Prevalence of chronic conditions and multimorbidities in a geographically defined geriatric population with diverse races and ethnicities. J Aging Health. 2018;30:421-444. doi:10.1177/0898264316680903

[7] Newman D, Levine E, Kishore SP. Prevalence of multiple chronic conditions in New York State, 2011-2016. PLoS One. 2019;14:e0211965. doi:10.1371/journal.pone.0211965

[8] Cheng C, Inder K, Chan SW. Coping with multiple chronic conditions: An integrative review. Nurs Health Sci. 2020;22(3):486-497. doi:10.1111/nhs.12695

[9] Sheridan PE, Mair CA, Quiñones AR. Associations between prevalent multimorbidity combinations and prospective disability and self-rated health among older adults in Europe. BMC Geriatr. 2019;19:198. doi:10.1186/s12877-019-1214-z

[10] Boersma P, Black LI, Ward BW. Prevalence of multiple chronic conditions among US adults, 2018. Prev Chronic Dis. 2020;17:E106. doi: 10.5888/pcd17.200130.

[11] Adams ML, Grandpre J, Katz DL, Shenson D. Linear association between number of modifiable risk factors and multiple chronic conditions: Results from the Behavioral Risk Factor Surveillance System. Prev Med. 2017;105:169-175. doi:10.1016/j.ypmed.2017.09.013

[12] McPhail SM. Multimorbidity in chronic disease: impact on health care resources and costs. Risk Manag Healthc Policy. 2016;9:143-56. doi: 10.2147/RMHP.S97248.

[13] Wang C, Kuo HC, Cheng SF, Hung JL, Xiong JH, Tang PL. Continuity of care and multiple chronic conditions impact frequent use of outpatient services. Health Informatics J. 2020;26(1):318-327. doi:10.1177/1460458218824720

[14] Adams ML. Differences between younger and older US adults with multiple chronic conditions. Prev Chronic Dis. 2017;14:E76. doi: 10.5888/pcd14.160613.

[15] Porter T, Ong BN, Sanders T. Living with multimorbidity?

The lived experience of multiple chronic conditions in later life. Health (London). 2020;24:701-718. doi:10.1177/1363459319834997

[16] Sturmberg JP, Bennett JM, Martin CM, Picard M. 'Multimorbidity' as the manifestation of network disturbances. J Eval Clin Pract. 2017;23:199-208. doi: 10.1111/jep.12587.

[17] Corwin EJ, Brewster G, Dunbar SB, Wells J, Hertzberg V, Holstad M, Song MK, Jones D. The metabolomic underpinnings of symptom burden in patients with multiple chronic conditions. Biol Res Nurs. 2020:1099800420958196. doi: 10.1177/1099800420958196.

[18] Pati S, Swain S, Knottnerus JA, Metsemakers JFM, van den Akker M. Health related quality of life in multimorbidity: a primary-care based study from Odisha, India. Health Qual Life Outcomes. 2019;17(1):116. doi:10.1186/s12955-019-1180-3

[19] Cheng C, Yang CY, Inder K, Chan SW. Illness perceptions, coping strategies, and quality of life in people with multiple chronic conditions. J Nurs Scholarsh. 2020;52:145-154. doi:10.1111/jnu.12540

[20] DuGoff EH, Canudas-Romo V, Buttorff C, Leff B, Anderson GF. Multiple chronic conditions and life expectancy: a life table analysis. Med Care. 2014;52:688-694. doi:10.1097/MLR.0000000000000166

[21] Wilson-Genderson M, Heid AR, Pruchno R. Onset of multiple chronic conditions and depressive symptoms: A life events perspective. Innov Aging. 2017;1:igx022. doi:10.1093/geroni/igx022

[22] Ge L, Ong R, Yap CW, Heng BH. Effects of chronic diseases on health-related quality of life and self-rated health among three adult age groups. Nurs Health Sci. 2019;21(2):214-222. doi:10.1111/nhs.12585

[23] Kadam UT, Roberts I, White S, et al. Conceptualizing multiple drug use in patients with comorbidity and multimorbidity: proposal for standard definitions beyond the term polypharmacy. J Clin Epidemiol. 2019;106:98-107. doi:10.1016/j.jclinepi.2018.10.014

[24] Laba TL, Cheng L, Kolhatkar A, Law MR. Cost-related nonadherence to medicines in people with multiple chronic conditions. Res Social Adm Pharm. 2020;16(3):415-421. doi:10.1016/j.sapharm.2019.06.008

[25] Guisado-Clavero M, Violán C, López-Jimenez T, et al. Medication patterns in older adults with multimorbidity: a cluster analysis of primary care patients. BMC Fam Pract. 2019;20:82. doi:10.1186/s12875-019-0969-9

[26] Falci L, Shi Z, Greenlee H. Multiple chronic conditions and use of complementary and alternative medicine among US adults: Results from the 2012 National Health Interview Survey. Prev Chronic Dis. 2016;13:E61. doi:10.5888/pcd13.150501

[27] Ouellet GM, Ouellet JA, Tinetti ME. Principle of rational prescribing and deprescribing in older adults with multiple chronic conditions. Ther Adv Drug Saf. 2018;9:639-652. doi:10.1177/2042098618791371

[28] Rahman FI, Aziz F, Huque S, Ether SA. Medication understanding and health literacy among patients with multiple chronic conditions: A study conducted in Bangladesh. J Public Health Res. 2020;9:1792. doi:10.4081/jphr.2020.1792

[29] Leppin AL, Montori VM, Gionfriddo MR. Minimally disruptive medicine: A pragmatically

comprehensive model for delivering care to patients with multiple chronic conditions. Healthcare (Basel). 2015;3:50-63. doi:10.3390/healthcare3010050

[30] Mihailoff M, Deb S, Lee JA, Lynn J. The effects of multiple chronic conditions on adult patient readmissions and hospital finances: A management case study. Inquiry. 2017;54:46958017729597. doi:10.1177/0046958017729597

[31] Tinetti ME, Green AR, Ouellet J, Rich MW, Boyd C. Caring for patients with multiple chronic conditions [published correction appears in Ann Intern Med. 2019 Mar 5;170(5):356]. Ann Intern Med. 2019;170(3):199-200. doi:10.7326/M18-3269

[32] Ploeg J, Canesi M, D Fraser K, McAiney C,Kaasalainen S, Maureen M-R, Sinead D, Garland Baird L,Chambers T. Experiences of community-dwelling older adults living with multiple chronic conditions: a qualitative study. BMJ Open. 2019;9(3):e023345. doi:10.1136/bmjopen-2018-023345

[33] González-Chica DA, Hill CL, Gill TK, Hay P, Haag D, Stocks N. Individual diseases or clustering of health conditions? Association between multiple chronic diseases and health-related quality of life in adults. Health Qual Life Outcomes. 2017;15(1):244. doi:10.1186/s12955-017-0806-6

[34] Egan BM, Sutherland SE, Tilkemeier PL, Davis RA, Rutledge V, Sinopoli A. A cluster-based approach for integrating clinical management of Medicare beneficiaries with multiple chronic conditions. PLoS One. 2019;14:e0217696. doi:10.1371/journal.pone.0217696

[35] Powell KR, Deroche C. Predictors and patterns of portal use in patients with multiple chronic conditions. Chronic Illn. 2020;16:275-283. doi:10.1177/1742395318803663

[36] Tinetti M, Dindo L, Smith CD, Blaum C, Costello D, Ouellet G, Rosen J, Hernandez-Bigos K, Geda M, Naik A. Challenges and strategies in patients' health priorities-aligned decision-making for older adults with multiple chronic conditions. PLoS One. 2019;14:e0218249. doi: 10.1371/journal.pone.0218249.

[37] Iglesias FH, Celada CA, Navarro CB, et al. Complex care needs in multiple chronic conditions: Population prevalence and characterization in primary care. A study protocol. Int J Integr Care. 2018;18:16. doi:10.5334/ijic.3292

[38] Boyd C, Smith CD, Masoudi FA, et al. Decision making for older adults with multiple chronic conditions: Executive summary for the American Geriatrics Society Guiding Principles on the care of older adults with multimorbidity. J Am Geriatr Soc. 2019;67(4):665-673. doi:10.1111/jgs.15809

[39] Zhang W, Radhakrishnan K. Evidence on selection, optimization, and compensation strategies to optimize aging with multiple chronic conditions: A literature review. Geriatr Nurs. 2018;39:534-542. doi:10.1016/j.gerinurse.2018.02.013

[40] Foo KM, Sundram M, Legido-Quigley H. Facilitators and barriers of managing patients with multiple chronic conditions in the community: a qualitative study. BMC Public Health. 2020;20(1):273. doi:10.1186/s12889-020-8375-8

[41] McGilton KS, Vellani S, Yeung L, et al. Identifying and understanding the health and social care needs of older adults with multiple chronic conditions and their caregivers: a scoping review. BMC Geriatr. 2018;18:231. doi:10.1186/s12877-018-0925-x

[42] Marengoni A, Fratiglioni L, Onder G. Improving public awareness of multimorbidity. J Am Med Dir Assoc. 2017;18:372-373. doi:10.1016/j.jamda.2017.01.010

[43] Riffin C, Van Ness PH, Iannone L, Fried T. Patient and caregiver perspectives on managing multiple health conditions. J Am Geriatr Soc. 2018;66:1992-1997. doi:10.1111/jgs.15501

[44] Bretos-Azcona PE, Sánchez-Iriso E, Cabasés Hita JM. Tailoring integrated care services for high-risk patients with multiple chronic conditions: a risk stratification approach using cluster analysis. BMC Health Serv Res. 2020;20(1):806. doi:10.1186/s12913-020-05668-7

[45] Sultan M, Kuluski K, McIsaac WJ, Cafazzo JA, Seto E. Turning challenges into design principles: Telemonitoring systems for patients with multiple chronic conditions. Health Informatics J. 2019;25:1188-1200. doi:10.1177/1460458217749882

Chapter 2

Exploring the Role of Rheumatic and Musculoskeletal Diseases in Multimorbidity

Daniela Simões and Raquel Lucas

Abstract

Non-communicable diseases (NCDs) frequently aggregate due to shared pathophysiological mechanisms, either as sequential steps in the same causal pathway or as common results of the same exposures, leading to a high prevalence of disease co-occurrence, a phenomenon known as multimorbidity. Multimorbidity is a patient-centered concept where all morbidities are regarded of equal importance irrespective of whether they started before or after any other disease in question. Rheumatic and musculoskeletal diseases (RMDs) are among the most prevalent groups of NCDs, and probably due to their high incidence and low case fatality, they are highly susceptible to multimorbidity. Complex patients, such as some of those with multimorbidity, are nowadays the norm, implying a growing concern that clinical practice guidelines fail to adequately address the care of complex patients. The ramifications of suffering from multimorbidity unfold for each patient, within their social, educational, cultural, behavioral, economic, and environmental contexts, which in turn affect disease management.

Keywords: rheumatic and musculoskeletal diseases, non-communicable diseases, multimorbidity, patient-centered care

1. Introduction

Multimorbidity is the concurrent presence of more than one chronic disease [1] in the same person and affects a substantial part of the adult population. Although the medical education and medical research are focused mainly on individual diseases, the study of multimorbidity is increasingly common. A recent bibliometric study revealed that the number of publications regarding this topic increased 60% after 2010 [2]. Nevertheless, the study of multimorbidity is still not sufficient to reduce the gap between the available evidence for single condition vs. multiple conditions [2].

Multimorbidity is a relatively new concept and a challenging area in clinical practice globally, and some confusion persists regarding its definition. For instance, the terminologies multimorbidity and comorbidity have been used interchangeably despite their differences. Comorbidity, as originally described by Feinstein in 1970 [3], is used to describe any clinical entity coexisting with an index disease under study. This term and its definition are widely accepted and used. However, the definition of multimorbidity, which is the term most frequently used when no index disease is designated, is still not consensual. Indeed, only in 2018, the term multimorbidity was accepted as a Medical Subject Heading (MeSH) by the United States National Library of Medicine and with the simple definition "the complex interactions of several co-existing diseases". Despite this somehow insufficient definition, it is usually accepted that multimorbidity takes into account chronic or long-term diseases or conditions, including both physical and mental diseases, with none considered the index disease [4].

Despite the stated differences, the concepts of comorbidity and multimorbidity are not mutually exclusive or contradictory, but consider a patient with more than one disease at the same time from different perspectives. While comorbidity considers any additional disease as consequence, complication, or coincidence, multimorbidity is a more generic, patient-centered concept, where all morbidities are regarded of equal importance irrespective of whether they started before or after any other disease in question, and that contemplates all aspects of a patient's condition, including potential disease interactions and potential pathophysiological links [5]. Multimorbidity considers that the pathophysiological links between these diseases, syndromes, or conditions may overlap and that their management may interact to varying degrees.

Highly prevalent chronic diseases, such as arthritis, diabetes, chronic lower respiratory tract disease, or stroke, are known to co-occur frequently [6], and even less prevalent conditions still may occur in the same person at the same time. It is clear that, at the population level, diseases may aggregate due to chance alone, i.e., the more frequent a disease is, the more likely it is to coexist with others even in the absence of a direct causal relation, particularly for conditions which become more common with increasing age. However, non-communicable diseases (NCDs) also frequently aggregate due to shared pathophysiological mechanisms, either as sequential steps in the same causal pathway (causal multimorbidity) or as common results of the same exposures (associative multimorbidity) [7]. One example is a known causal pathway between rheumatoid arthritis and cardiovascular disease [8]. Another example is the increased risk of both osteoarthritis and type 2 diabetes in people with obesity, a shared risk factor between several NCDs that consequently increases the likelihood of these diseases clustering in the same subject [9]. This framework provides a causal or associative meaning to several mechanisms commonly used to explain for disease co-occurrence: general disease susceptibility, interaction between gene and environment, association between morbidities in a mutually reinforcing causal loop, effects on different organs of psychosocial and cultural factors, life events and coping styles, and common underlying pathogenic mechanisms, such as chronic inflammation [7, 10].

2. Multimorbidity burden

Multimorbidity is becoming increasingly important in research and daily clinical practice. Its burden to both the individual and society is increasing, probably due to higher life expectancy, lowered thresholds for diagnoses, advances in medical care, and possibly due to a true increase in the prevalence of some chronic diseases [11]. Despite the existence of abundant information regarding epidemiology, risk factors, and management of individual chronic diseases, for multimorbidity only a few clinical guidelines exist making informed decisions harder. For example, following clinical practice guidelines for individual chronic conditions, a recent systematic review reported that a hypothetical 78-year-old woman with five chronic conditions [osteoporosis, osteoarthritis, diabetes type 2, hypertension, and chronic obstructive pulmonary disease (COPD)] would be prescribed up to 12 separate medications, taken at five times during the day, and should be engaged in

14 non-pharmacological activities [12, 13]. Given that each one of these diseases has different therapies, the management strategy for the patient with multimorbidity may be influenced by the care provided to each one of the conditions, including limitations of life expectancy, interactions between therapies, and/or contraindications to therapy for one condition due to other conditions [14]. Additionally, most times, the use of many services to manage individual diseases can become duplicative and inefficient and may be burdensome and unsafe for patients because of poor coordination and integration. In fact, a key aspect of multimorbidity is that chronic diseases are likely to act synergistically [15], causing an overall burden that can be larger than the sum of their individual impacts.

At the patient level, multimorbidity is associated with higher mortality [16], worsened functional status, and poorer quality of life [17]. Additionally, people living with multimorbidity have greater self-care needs [18] and are especially likely to rely on a caregiver for health management [19]. At the healthcare level, it implies increased risk of receiving less than best practice care [20], more frequent postoperative complications [21], longer hospitalization, higher likelihood of readmission [22], more frequent healthcare utilization, higher direct costs [23, 24], and increased use of polypharmacy with the potential for adverse drug effects [25]. With all these adverse health outcomes, the ramifications of suffering from multimorbidity affect the individual within social, educational, cultural, behavioral, economic, and environmental circumstances, which in turn affect disease management.

Studies have shown that age, household income, and family structure are the most important measured predictors of the multimorbidity status [26]. Moreover, multimorbidity tends to be more common in females than in males [26, 27]. The presence of multimorbidity also suggests higher risk of additional conditions, i.e., people with multimorbidity are at a higher risk of being diagnosed with two or more new diseases than those with no disease [28], probably due to increased interaction with healthcare professionals and higher healthcare utilization. Additionally, several important modifiable risk factors that are associated with the development of individual chronic diseases may play an important role in multimorbidity. These include lifestyle factors such as tobacco smoking and alcohol intake, over- and undernutrition, physical inactivity, and occupational exposures [29–32]. Many of these factors are common to multiple diseases. For instance, smoking increases the risk of chronic respiratory diseases, cardiovascular diseases, and neoplasms, while obesity increases the risk of cardiovascular diseases and musculoskeletal disorders. Therefore, it is not surprising that the presence of these risk factors increases the risk of a particular combination of chronic diseases. A recent bibliometric study showed that the risk factors most commonly mentioned in multimorbidity studies are physical activity and obesity/high body mass index [2]. Additionally, a recent overview of systematic reviews summarized the evidence on risk factors for multimorbidity into four groups: biomedical and individual factors (aging, women, high number of previous diseases, negative life events, external health locus of control, and mental disorders), health behaviors (smoking, overweight, obesity, high waist to hip ratio, and low physical activity), socioeconomic characteristics (lower social economic status, lower education, less social networks, full dependency, and unemployment), and social and environmental factors (living in urban areas in lower middle income country) [33].

Despite the increase in research outputs regarding multimorbidity, the evaluation of the burden of multimorbidity and its population impact remains challenging. In the European Union, there are an estimated 50 million people with multimorbidity, and this number is expected to grow as the population ages [34]. Estimates of the prevalence of multimorbidity vary from 4.4% to over 90% [35–37], a discrepancy driven by distinct study populations or data sources, usually involving differences in demographic characteristics and disease types or classification. Despite this, up to the present, no gold standard exists regarding how to assess multimorbidity, and there is no consensus on which conditions should be considered or on the method used for measuring multimorbidity, which makes comparisons among studies difficult.

3. The role of rheumatic and musculoskeletal diseases in multimorbidity

Rheumatic and musculoskeletal diseases (RMDs) are among the most prevalent groups of NCDs [38]. They are strong determinants of pain [39] and disability [40] and the first to third largest contributors to years lived with disability (YLDs) in almost all world regions [41]. Additionally, they have a high impact on quality of life [42], complexity of medication regimens [43], and affect the ability to continue paid employment [44]. Due to their high incidence and low case fatality, RMDs frequently co-exist with other conditions [37, 45]. Despite their well-known association with a wide scope of adverse health outcomes [46–49], the inclusion of RMDs in multimorbidity research tends to be inconsistent and selective. However, evidence supports that RMDs appear to form a principal component of certain multimorbidity clusters [50] and are common in multimorbidity [51, 52], with one study reporting that even after adjustment for age and gender, the odds of multimorbidity were greater in respondents with musculoskeletal conditions than those with any of the non-musculoskeletal conditions included in different definitions of multimorbidity assessed [51].

RMDs are also a highly heterogeneous group of NCDs [38], from inflammatory rheumatic diseases (such as rheumatoid arthritis and spondyloarthritis) to degenerative conditions (such as osteoarthritis), fragility conditions (such as osteoporosis), or regional pain syndromes (such as low back pain, neck pain and, the chronic widespread pain syndrome) [53]. RMDs are common throughout the life course, but some become even more common at older ages, in particular osteoarthritis. Despite this, RMDs are not always assessed in multimorbidity studies, and when assessed, they are usually restricted to osteoarthritis [54] or to broadly encapsulating categories that include arthritis, other joint disorders, or other painful conditions in the same category [26, 55].

It is plausible that the prevalence of multimorbidity might vary for subtypes of RMDs included in each definition. The subgroups with the highest prevalence of multimorbidity are typically osteoporosis, osteoarthritis, and inflammatory arthritis [51], but it remains to be determined whether RMDs in general, or only particular subgroups of RMDs, are associated with increased prevalence of multimorbidity.

Furthermore, multimorbidity research typically focuses on older people, naturally excluding generally less disabling RMDs, such as work-related musculoskeletal conditions. However, multimorbidity is not simply a process of aging [36], suggesting that to fully capture the burden of RMDs in multimorbidity a broader age range should be evaluated. As a matter of fact, considering that the presence of one condition increases the risk of multimorbidity in disease-specific populations (probably due to shared lifestyle and biomedical disease risk factors, as well as medication use [56] or iatrogenic effects [57]), the study of the role of RMDs in multimorbidity should start at young ages to fully capture the heterogeneity of RMDs, including soft tissue disorders or others that start at younger working ages.

Many important risk factors for common RMDs show remarkable overlap with risk factors for multimorbidity. For example, age and female gender are two of the most important non-modifiable risk factors for some RMDs [58], and as previously stated, they are also common risk factors for multimorbidity. Modifiable risk factors such as obesity or low physical activity are importantly associated with osteoarthritis and regional pain syndromes, including low back pain [59]. Additionally, smoking is the main modifiable risk factor for inflammatory arthritis, and smoking, poor nutrition, and low physical activity are lifestyle risk factors for osteoporosis [60]. All these risk factors have been linked to multimorbidity in recent publications [29–32].

Because of the heterogeneous multimorbidity definitions used in different studies, it is difficult to fully assess the impact of RMDs on multimorbidity. However, RMDs usually aggregate with a wide set of NCDs. An Australian systematic review of population-based studies in the elderly found that over 50% of elderly patients with arthritis also had hypertension followed by cardiovascular diseases, dyslipidemia, diabetes, and mental health problems, whereas 60% of elderly patients with asthma reported arthritis followed by cardiovascular diseases and diabetes [61]. According to several systematic reviews, arthritis or osteoarthritis is usually comorbid with hypertension, cardiovascular diseases, dyslipidemia, diabetes, mental health problems, asthma, depression, and metabolic conditions [45, 61–63].

As previously described [64–66], RMDs frequently cluster with cardiometabolic conditions due to common pathophysiological risk factors, such as immobility, obesity, and systemic inflammation [67]. Additionally, pleuropulmonary disease may occur in patients with systemic autoimmune rheumatic diseases due to several causes, including infection in the treated patient, toxic medication reactions, and inherent manifestations of the diseases themselves [68]. Also, studies have shown a slightly increased risk of specific malignancies in people with rheumatoid arthritis [69], possibly due to smoking as a common risk factor for rheumatoid arthritis and lung cancer [70] and estrogen changes, which are common to rheumatoid arthritis and breast cancer [71]. A strong bidirectional relation between depressive states and musculoskeletal symptoms, especially pain, is well documented, which accounts for the clustering of these conditions [72]. These findings can be interpreted in the light of the current discussion about inflammatory as well as oxidative and nitrosative stress pathways that underpin the common pathophysiology of depression and RMDs [73]. Additionally, inflammatory cytokines, glucocorticoid treatment, immobilization, and reduced physical activity due to tender joints and muscle weakness have shown to play a key role in favoring low bone mineral density in RMDs [74], especially in people with rheumatoid arthritis [75].

The specific combination of RMDs with other NCDs also seems to have a strongly deleterious effect in adverse health outcomes. For example, co-occurrence of pulmonary and cardiac diseases is most often associated with mortality, but work disability is more strongly associated with depression [76]. Therefore, when trying to assess how multimorbidity affects prognosis, we need to define which disease combinations we are referring to and which outcome is of greatest interest. Slater and colleagues [77] found that among people with diabetes, cardiovascular, and respiratory diseases, comorbid musculoskeletal conditions increased the risk and accounted for a substantial proportion of activity limitations. Also, patients with rheumatoid arthritis and comorbidities are less likely to achieve treatment targets such as remission or low disease activity [78]. Others demonstrated that multimorbidity and depressive symptoms are strongly linked to functional limitations and lower self-rated health [79], that RMDs in multimorbidity worsen daily functioning and quality of life [17], and that multimorbidity is associated with frequent healthcare utilization and higher costs for the healthcare system [80]. Depression seems to interact synergistically with arthritis and neck/back disorders to increase the odds of reporting chronic pain beyond an additive model [81]. Additionally, the presence of RMDs in the context of multimorbidity tends to amplify the risk of adverse work outcomes and especially of sick leave [52].

4. The challenges of multimorbidity management

The management of patients with multimorbidity is challenging. Although it could be expected that people with multimorbidity might be receiving better quality of healthcare than that individuals with only one disorder, at least partly because of greater contact with healthcare services [82], people with multimorbidity have more difficulties with disintegration of care, polypharmacy, and medical error because much specialized care is focused on the treatment of one disease [5]. Those with multimorbidity frequently receive care from family physicians, other medical specialists, and other healthcare professionals, such as nurses or physiotherapists, who may not be communicating effectively with each other [83]. Additionally, and despite the confirmed effectiveness of many individual treatments commonly used in chronic conditions, each additional therapy carries an additional burden, known as treatment burden, which includes physical effects of treatment, financial losses, and the psychosocial effects of time demands and dependence on others for assistance [84]. This means that people often suffer from a combination of disease and treatment burdens and that people receiving multiple treatments will have a higher treatment burden than those receiving only one treatment.

Currently, the main challenge of health professionals when targeting multimorbidity is to try to step aside from a disease-centered perspective, very deeply rooted in health professionals' education and strongly encouraged through pay-for-performance systems, to switch to the patient as the focus of treatment. For example, the typical treatment perspective for a patient with RMDs and other conditions focuses on the comorbidity concept, i.e., in the treatment of the index disease [5]. A medical doctor, usually a rheumatologist, will apply the treat-to-target concept to induce remission of that disease [85], hoping that this treatment will also positively affect non-RMD comorbidities. The treat-to-target approach is generally defined as a proactive treatment strategy, operationalized as a precise treatment algorithm, in which the clinician treats the patient aggressively enough to reach and maintain specific goals, such as remission or low disease activity [85]. In contrast, when considering the multimorbidity concept, the focus is on treating the patient, usually trying to improve overall well-being. In multimorbidity, it is harder to assess treatment effectiveness, and other concepts such as quality of life, overall function or health, and the patients' preferences should be also considered [5]. In order to help the clinicians, a recent clinical guideline suggesting a patient-centered approach to multimorbidity was published [86, 87]. It is important to notice that it is very difficult to publish guidelines concerning a disease-centered treatment for every combination of chronic conditions, which is one of the reasons why multimorbidity guidelines are more likely to take a patient-centered approach, targeting general well-being, quality of life, independence, autonomy, and improved function, but especially patient's goals, values, and priorities [86]. By implementing the concept of patient-centered care in daily practice, a greater effectiveness of diagnosis and treatment approaches and also improved clinical outcomes are expected.

This new clinical guideline suggests that in patient-centered care it is important to understand the patient's life, establishing what is important to them, and acknowledge the current disease and treatment burdens. After that, a revision of the patient's current medicines and other treatments should be done. The risks and benefits of each treatment (including non-pharmacological ones) should be weighted, and later, an individualized management plan, including timing of follow-up, should be developed and agreed upon with the patient [86]. Health professionals will have the most difficult task: to balance medical knowledge and expertise with patients' goals, when trying to reduce the impact of any conditions on the adverse health outcomes that really worry the patient. It is not only about attaining one disease remission but rather to achieve a "healthy" life, and this is even more important when the patient is chronically ill.

Patient-centered care for patients with multimorbidity can be described as a care which (1) is attentive to patient's psychosocial as well as physical needs, (2) explores the patient's concerns and priorities for care, (3) conveys a sense of partnership between the patient and physician, (4) facilitates active patient involvement in decision-making, and (5) is coordinated across professionals, facilities, and support systems [88, 89]. However, the evidence regarding the effectiveness of such care is still lacking. The need for such evidence, including the need for patient care guidelines and health programs that are multiple disease-centered, is nowadays well established. Despite the recent publication of new guidelines and frameworks regarding patient-centered and integrated care [90, 91], the implementation of these recommendations in day-to-day work will require a re-organization in the way care is delivered. In a qualitative study, Bayliss and colleagues [18] explored the healthcare priorities of patients with multimorbidity. The priorities for patients were easy access to care and clinicians, but especially they desired healthcare providers who had a caring attitude and listened to them, understanding that their needs were unique and fluctuating. A recent systematic review [92] described comprehensive care programs targeting multimorbidity patients and estimated their effectiveness regarding improvement of patient- and caregiver-related outcomes, healthcare utilization, and costs. The authors concluded that providing comprehensive care might result in higher patient satisfaction, less depressive symptoms, a better health-related quality of life, or functioning, but also found that the evidence is still insufficient. More (good quality) studies using more appropriate outcome measures are needed [92].

Patient-centered care must be provided by a multidisciplinary team, and this is a great challenge. There must be clarity about who will be responsible for carrying out the different actions outlined in a plan, with appropriate support and coordination between professionals. Although it would be expected that several health professionals would have expertise in assessment and management of RMDs and differ mainly by the types of interventions they use, this is often not the case, given that different professionals have different curricula and often different perspectives regarding diseases and treatment goals [93]. So, it should be recognized that an integrated approach with all the disciplines and professionals working together is the ideal way of achieving the best outcome for the patient. Healthcare services should be aware of this paradigm shift and must provide integrated coordinated multidisciplinary care; however, this is a multifaceted challenge that cannot be overcome with a single effort.

5. Conclusion

Complex patients, such as some of those with multimorbidity, are nowadays the norm, implying a growing concern that clinical practice guidelines fail to adequately address the care of complex patients. As already mentioned, the ramifications of suffering from multimorbidity unfold for each patient, within their social, educational, cultural, behavioral, economic, and environmental contexts, which in turn affect disease management. The healthcare system in several countries is typically guided by clinical practice guidelines that are oriented toward single disease [94]. This poses a challenge for primary care professionals who try to implement evidence from these guidelines in patients with multimorbidity. As described by Duffield and colleagues [53], people with multimorbidity are often required to carry out numerous tasks to maintain their health. The responsibilities listed by the authors include managing different tablets to be taken at specific times of day, week, or only occasionally; keeping stock of their pills, creams, inhalers, and injections; requesting repeat prescriptions on time; visiting the pharmacy to collect items; performing non-pharmacological treatments such as physiotherapy or other complementary interventions; and monitoring treatment effectiveness with regular lab analyses, physical tests, and medical appointments [53]. The time and effort required to remember and attend these appointments, including travel time, may require an additional treatment burden placed upon the individual [84]. Having a RMD as part of multimorbidity makes all of these activities even more difficult. People with arthritis report great difficulty or inability to grasp small objects; reach above one's head; sit more than 2 hours; lift or carry 10 pounds; climb a flight of stairs; push a heavy object; walk a 1/4 mile; stand for more than 2 hours; and stoop, bend, or kneel [95]. As a result of restricted mobility and function, having a RMD can hamper the execution of many of the tasks required in multimorbidity care, limiting people's ability to manage their health.

The impact of RMDs on patients and society should be acknowledged, as they are mostly non-fatal conditions with great effects at older ages. Regardless of the multimorbidity definition applied, musculoskeletal conditions are a common component of multimorbidity [51], and most working-age adults who met the definition of multimorbidity had a musculoskeletal condition [96]. This is an important finding because the strategies to include and classify musculoskeletal conditions within multimorbidity research have been inconsistent. Policy makers and public health teams should be aware of the importance of musculoskeletal health. Frequently, osteoarthritis and osteoporosis are seen as a natural consequence of aging and back pain as normal in working ages. The importance of early appropriate treatment for many musculoskeletal conditions in order to prevent chronicity and to reduce disability is undervalued. Often, adherence to treatment plans is less than optimal since patients are typically given little information about their condition; and many have misconceptions about treatments [97]. However, it is important to understand that even if the condition itself cannot be suppressed, health professionals can contribute to improve the patient's general well-being, quality of life, independence, autonomy, and general function.

Governments and public health teams along with healthcare stakeholders should take multimorbidity into account when designing, implementing, and evaluating public health education, programmes, and campaigns. They should identify and understand the needs and requirements of people living with multimorbidity (and with RMDs in particular) in their populations. They should also identify, prioritize, and target adverse health outcomes. They should acknowledge that targeting risk factors can potentially reduce the burden of multimorbidity in the long term. It is time to face multimorbidity.

In conclusion, although population aging has been a remarkable achievement of public health and clinical medicine, it poses great challenges that can only be overcome if clinicians, researchers, and policy makers are aware of the complexity of multimorbidity, which needs specialization, but also a holistic approach to ensure that patients receive coordinated care. However, more studies on RMDs and multimorbidity are still needed. Further evidence may help to better understand reasons for poorer health in certain groups and to aid their disease management. It may also contribute to assess the effect of multimorbidity on long-term outcomes, to identify prognostic factors, to develop effective interventions, and to support integrated patient-centered care programmes.

Conflict of interest

All authors have declared that no conflict of interest exists.

Author details

Daniela Simões[1,2]* and Raquel Lucas[1,3]

1 EPIUnit—Instituto de Saúde Pública, Universidade do Porto, Porto, Portugal

2 Escola Superior de Saúde de Santa Maria, Porto, Portugal

3 Departamento de Ciências da Saúde Pública e Forenses e Educação Médica, Faculdade de Medicina, Universidade do Porto, Porto, Portugal

*Address all correspondence to: daniela.simoes@ispup.up.pt

References

[1] Valderas JM, Starfield B, Sibbald B, Salisbury C, Roland M. Defining comorbidity: Implications for understanding health and health services. Annals of Family Medicine. 2009;**7**(4):357-363

[2] Xu X, Mishra GD, Jones M. Mapping the global research landscape and knowledge gaps on multimorbidity: A bibliometric study. Journal of Global Health. 2017;**7**(1):010414

[3] Feinstein AR. The pre-therapeutic classification of co-morbidity in chronic disease. Journal of Chronic Diseases. 1970;**23**(7):455-468

[4] Almirall J, Fortin M. The coexistence of terms to describe the presence of multiple concurrent diseases. Journal of Comorbidity. 2013;**3**:4-9

[5] Radner H, Yoshida K, Smolen JS, Solomon DH. Multimorbidity and rheumatic conditions-enhancing the concept of comorbidity. Nature Reviews Rheumatology. 2014;**10**(4):252-256

[6] Weiss CO, Boyd CM, Yu Q, Wolff JL, Leff B. Patterns of prevalent major chronic disease among older adults in the United States. Journal of the American Medical Association. 2007;**298**(10):1160-1162

[7] Marengoni A, Fratiglioni L. Disease clusters in older adults: Rationale and need for investigation. Journal of the American Geriatrics Society. 2011;**59**(12):2395-2396

[8] Meune C, Touze E, Trinquart L, Allanore Y. Trends in cardiovascular mortality in patients with rheumatoid arthritis over 50 years: A systematic review and meta-analysis of cohort studies. Rheumatology. 2009;**48**(10):1309-1313

[9] Duclos M. Osteoarthritis, obesity and type 2 diabetes: The weight of waist circumference. Annals of Physical and Rehabilitation Medicine. 2016;**59**(3):157-160

[10] Rhee SH, Hewitt JK, Corley RP, Willcutt EG, Pennington BF. Testing hypotheses regarding the causes of comorbidity: Examining the underlying deficits of comorbid disorders. Journal of Abnormal Psychology. 2005;**114**(3):346-362

[11] Starfield B. Challenges to primary care from co- and multi-morbidity. Primary Health Care Research & Development. 2011;**12**(1):1-2

[12] Boyd CM, Darer J, Boult C, Fried LP, Boult L, Wu AW. Clinical practice guidelines and quality of care for older patients with multiple comorbid diseases: Implications for pay for performance. Journal of the American Medical Association. 2005;**294**(6):716-724

[13] Buffel du Vaure C, Ravaud P, Baron G, Barnes C, Gilberg S, Boutron I. Potential workload in applying clinical practice guidelines for patients with chronic conditions and multimorbidity: A systematic analysis. BMJ Open. 2016;**6**(3):e010119

[14] Safford MM, Allison JJ, Kiefe CI. Patient complexity: More than comorbidity. The vector model of complexity. Journal of General Internal Medicine. 2007;**22**(Suppl 3):382-390

[15] Rijken M, van Kerkhof M, Dekker J, Schellevis FG. Comorbidity of chronic diseases: Effects of disease pairs on physical and mental functioning. Quality of Life Research. 2005;**14**(1):45-55

[16] Menotti A, Mulder I, Nissinen A, Giampaoli S, Feskens EJM, Kromhout D. Prevalence of morbidity and multimorbidity in elderly male populations

and their impact on 10-year all-cause mortality: The FINE study (Finland, Italy, Netherlands, Elderly). Journal of Clinical Epidemiology. 2001;**54**(7):680-686

[17] Loza E, Jover JA, Rodriguez L, Carmona L. Multimorbidity: Prevalence, effect on quality of life and daily functioning, and variation of this effect when one condition is a rheumatic disease. Seminars in Arthritis and Rheumatism. 2009;**38**(4):312-319

[18] Bayliss EA, Edwards AE, Steiner JF, Main DS. Processes of care desired by elderly patients with multimorbidities. Family Practice. 2008;**25**(4):287-293

[19] Wolff JL, Roter DL. Hidden in plain sight: Medical visit companions as a resource for vulnerable older adults. Archives of Internal Medicine. 2008;**168**(13):1409-1415

[20] Vogeli C, Shields AE, Lee TA, Gibson TB, Marder WD, Weiss KB, et al. Multiple chronic conditions: Prevalence, health consequences, and implications for quality, care management, and costs. Journal of General Internal Medicine. 2007;**22**(Suppl 3):391-395

[21] Greenfield S, Apolone G, McNeil BJ, Cleary PD. The importance of co-existent disease in the occurrence of postoperative complications and one-year recovery in patients undergoing total hip replacement. Comorbidity and outcomes after hip replacement. Medical Care. 1993;**31**(2):141-154

[22] Librero J, Peiro S, Ordinana R. Chronic comorbidity and outcomes of hospital care: Length of stay, mortality, and readmission at 30 and 365 days. Journal of Clinical Epidemiology. 1999;**52**(3):171-179

[23] Wolff JL, Starfield B, Anderson G. Prevalence, expenditures, and complications of multiple chronic conditions in the elderly. Archives of Internal Medicine. 2002;**162**(20):2269-2276

[24] Simões D, Araujo FA, Monjardino T, Severo M, Cruz I, Carmona L, et al. The population impact of rheumatic and musculoskeletal diseases in relation to other non-communicable disorders: Comparing two estimation approaches. Rheumatology International. 2018;**38**(5):905-915

[25] Condelius A, Edberg AK, Jakobsson U, Hallberg IR. Hospital admissions among people 65+ related to multimorbidity, municipal and outpatient care. Archives of Gerontology and Geriatrics. 2008;**46**(1):41-55

[26] Agborsangaya CB, Lau D, Lahtinen M, Cooke T, Johnson JA. Multimorbidity prevalence and patterns across socioeconomic determinants: A cross-sectional survey. BMC Public Health. 2012;**12**:201

[27] Fortin M, Hudon C, Haggerty J, Akker M, Almirall J. Prevalence estimates of multimorbidity: A comparative study of two sources. BMC Health Services Research. 2010;**10**:111

[28] Satariano WA, Ragland DR. The effect of comorbidity on 3-year survival of women with primary breast cancer. Annals of Internal Medicine. 1994;**120**(2):104-110

[29] Divo MJ, Martinez CH, Mannino DM. Ageing and the epidemiology of multimorbidity. The European Respiratory Journal. 2014;**44**(4):1055-1068

[30] Agborsangaya CB, Ngwakongnwi E, Lahtinen M, Cooke T, Johnson JA. Multimorbidity prevalence in the general population: The role of obesity in chronic disease clustering. BMC Public Health. 2013;**13**:1161

[31] Autenrieth CS, Kirchberger I, Heier M, Zimmermann AK, Peters A, Doring A, et al. Physical activity is inversely associated with multimorbidity in elderly men: Results from the

KORA-Age Augsburg Study. Preventive Medicine. 2013;**57**(1):17-19

[32] Dhalwani NN, O'Donovan G, Zaccardi F, Hamer M, Yates T, Davies M, et al. Long terms trends of multimorbidity and association with physical activity in older English population. International Journal of Behavioral Nutrition and Physical Activity. 2016;**13**:8

[33] Xu X, Mishra GD, Jones M. Evidence on multimorbidity from definition to intervention: An overview of systematic reviews. Ageing Research Reviews. 2017;**37**:53-68

[34] Rijken M, Struckmann V, Dyakova M, Melchiorre MG, Rissanen S, van Ginneken E, et al. ICARE4EU: Improving care for people with multiple chronic conditions in Europe. Eurohealth. 2013;**19**(3):29-31

[35] Fortin M, Bravo G, Hudon C, Vanasse A, Lapointe L. Prevalence of multimorbidity among adults seen in family practice. Annals of Family Medicine. 2005;**3**(3):223-228

[36] Taylor AW, Price K, Gill TK, Adams R, Pilkington R, Carrangis N, et al. Multimorbidity—Not just an older person's issue. Results from an Australian biomedical study. BMC Public Health. 2010;**10**:718

[37] Violan C, Foguet-Boreu Q, Flores-Mateo G, Salisbury C, Blom J, Freitag M, et al. Prevalence, determinants and patterns of multimorbidity in primary care: A systematic review of observational studies. PLoS One. 2014;**9**(7):e102149

[38] Woolf AD, Vos T, March L. How to measure the impact of musculoskeletal conditions. Best Practice & Research. Clinical Rheumatology. 2010;**24**(6):723-732

[39] WHO. The burden of musculoskeletal conditions at the start of the new millenium. World Health Organization Technical Report Series. 2003;**919**:1-218

[40] CDC. Prevalence and most common causes of disability among adults—United States, 2005. MMWR. Morbidity and Mortality Weekly Report. 2009;**58**(16):421-426

[41] Vos T. Years lived with disability (YLDs) for 1160 sequelae of 289 diseases and injuries 1990-2010: A systematic analysis for the Global Burden of Disease Study. Lancet. 2010;**380**(9859):2163-2196

[42] Alonso J, Ferrer M, Gandek B, Ware JE Jr, Aaronson NK, Mosconi P, et al. Health-related quality of life associated with chronic conditions in eight countries: Results from the international quality of life assessment (IQOLA) project. Quality of Life Research. 2004;**13**(2):283-298

[43] Manias E, Claydon-Platt K, McColl GJ, Bucknall TK, Brand CA. Managing complex medication regimens: Perspectives of consumers with osteoarthritis and healthcare professionals. The Annals of Pharmacotherapy. 2007;**41**(5):764-771

[44] Burton W, Morrison A, Maclean R, Ruderman E. Systematic review of studies of productivity loss due to rheumatoid arthritis. Occupational Medicine. 2006;**56**(1):18-27

[45] Diederichs C, Berger K, Bartels DB. The measurement of multiple chronic diseases—A systematic review on existing multimorbidity indices. The Journals of Gerontology. Series A, Biological Sciences and Medical Sciences. 2011;**66**(3):301-311

[46] Perruccio AV, Power JD, Badley EM. The relative impact of 13 chronic conditions across three different outcomes. Journal of Epidemiology and Community Health. 2007;**61**(12): 1056-1061

[47] Palazzo C, Ravaud JF, Trinquart L, Dalichampt M, Ravaud P, Poiraudeau S. Respective contribution of chronic conditions to disability in France: Results from the national disability-health survey. PLoS One. 2012;7(9):e44994

[48] Molarius A, Janson S. Self-rated health, chronic diseases, and symptoms among middle-aged and elderly men and women. Journal of Clinical Epidemiology. 2002;**55**(4):364-370

[49] Griffith L, Raina P, Wu H, Zhu B, Stathokostas L. Population attributable risk for functional disability associated with chronic conditions in Canadian older adults. Age and Ageing. 2010;**39**(6):738-745

[50] Prados-Torres A, Calderon-Larranaga A, Hancco-Saavedra J, Poblador-Plou B, van den Akker M. Multimorbidity patterns: A systematic review. Journal of Clinical Epidemiology. 2014;**67**(3):254-266

[51] Lowe DB, Taylor MJ, Hill SJ. Cross-sectional examination of musculoskeletal conditions and multimorbidity: Influence of different thresholds and definitions on prevalence and association estimates. BMC Research Notes. 2017;**10**(1):51

[52] van der Zee-Neuen A, Putrik P, Ramiro S, Keszei A, de Bie R, Chorus A, et al. Work outcome in persons with musculoskeletal diseases: Comparison with other chronic diseases & the role of musculoskeletal diseases in multimorbidity. BMC Musculoskeletal Disorders. 2017;**18**(1):10

[53] Duffield SJ, Ellis BM, Goodson N, Walker-Bone K, Conaghan PG, Margham T, et al. The contribution of musculoskeletal disorders in multimorbidity: Implications for practice and policy. Best Practice & Research. Clinical Rheumatology. 2017;**31**(2):129-144

[54] Kadam UT, Croft PR. Clinical comorbidity in osteoarthritis: Associations with physical function in older patients in family practice. The Journal of Rheumatology. 2007;**34**(9):1899-1904

[55] Barnett K, Mercer SW, Norbury M, Watt G, Wyke S, Guthrie B. Epidemiology of multimorbidity and implications for health care, research, and medical education: A cross-sectional study. Lancet. 2012;**380**(9836):37-43

[56] Roberts ER, Green D, Kadam UT. Chronic condition comorbidity and multidrug therapy in general practice populations: A cross-sectional linkage study. BMJ Open. 2014;**4**(7):e005429

[57] Offidani E, Fava GA, Sonino N. Iatrogenic comorbidity in childhood and adolescence: New insights from the use of antidepressant drugs. CNS Drugs. 2014;**28**(9):769-774

[58] Lawrence RC, Helmick CG, Arnett FC, Deyo RA, Felson DT, Giannini EH, et al. Estimates of the prevalence of arthritis and selected musculoskeletal disorders in the United States. Arthritis and Rheumatism. 1998;**41**(5):778-799

[59] Coggon D, Reading I, Croft P, McLaren M, Barrett D, Cooper C. Knee osteoarthritis and obesity. International Journal of Obesity and Related Metabolic Disorders. 2001;**25**(5):622-627

[60] Clark PM, Ellis BM. A public health approach to musculoskeletal health. Best Practice & Research. Clinical Rheumatology. 2014;**28**(3):517-532

[61] Caughey GE, Vitry AI, Gilbert AL, Roughead EE. Prevalence of comorbidity of chronic diseases in Australia. BMC Public Health. 2008;**8**:221

[62] Willadsen TG, Bebe A, Koster-Rasmussen R, Jarbol DE, Guassora AD, Waldorff FB, et al. The role of diseases,

risk factors and symptoms in the definition of multimorbidity—A systematic review. Scandinavian Journal of Primary Health Care. 2016;**34**(2):112-121

[63] Sinnige J, Braspenning J, Schellevis F, Stirbu-Wagner I, Westert G, Korevaar J. The prevalence of disease clusters in older adults with multiple chronic diseases—A systematic literature review. PLoS One. 2013;**8**(11):e79641

[64] Holden L, Scuffham PA, Hilton MF, Muspratt A, Ng SK, Whiteford HA. Patterns of multimorbidity in working Australians. Population Health Metrics. 2011;**9**:15

[65] Freund T, Kunz CU, Ose D, Szecsenyi J, Peters-Klimm F. Patterns of multimorbidity in primary care patients at high risk of future hospitalization. Population Health Management. 2012;**15**(2):119-124

[66] Simões D, Araújo FA, Severo M, Monjardino T, Cruz I, Carmona L, et al. Patterns and consequences of multimorbidity in the general population: There is no chronic disease management without rheumatic disease management. Arthritis Care and Research. 2017;**69**(1):12-20

[67] Meek IL, Picavet HS, Vonkeman HE, Verschuren WM, van de Laar MA. Increased cardiovascular risk factors in different rheumatic diseases compared with the general population. Rheumatology. 2013;**52**(1):210-216

[68] Schneider F, Gruden J, Tazelaar HD, Leslie KO. Pleuropulmonary pathology in patients with rheumatic disease. Archives of Pathology & Laboratory Medicine. 2012;**136**(10):1242-1252

[69] Simon TA, Thompson A, Gandhi KK, Hochberg MC, Suissa S. Incidence of malignancy in adult patients with rheumatoid arthritis: A meta-analysis. Arthritis Research & Therapy. 2015;**17**:212

[70] Sugiyama D, Nishimura K, Tamaki G, Tsuji T, Nakazawa A, Morinobu S, et al. Impact of smoking as a risk factor for developing rheumatoid arthritis: A meta-analysis of observational studies. Annals of the Rheumatic Diseases. 2010;**69**(1):70-81

[71] James WH. Hypothesis: Gonadal hormones act as confounders in epidemiological studies of the associations between some behavioural risk factors and some pathological conditions. Journal of Theoretical Biology. 2001;**209**(1):97-102

[72] Bair MJ, Robinson RL, Katon W, Kroenke K. Depression and pain comorbidity: A literature review. Archives of Internal Medicine. 2003;**163**(20):2433-2445

[73] Maes M, Kubera M, Obuchowiczwa E, Goehler L, Brzeszcz J. Depression's multiple comorbidities explained by (neuro)inflammatory and oxidative & nitrosative stress pathways. Neuro Endocrinology Letters. 2011;**32**(1):7-24

[74] Maruotti N, Corrado A, Cantatore FP. Osteoporosis and rheumatic diseases. Reumatismo. 2014;**66**(2):125-135

[75] van Staa TP, Geusens P, Bijlsma JW, Leufkens HG, Cooper C. Clinical assessment of the long-term risk of fracture in patients with rheumatoid arthritis. Arthritis and Rheumatism. 2006;**54**(10):3104-3112

[76] Gabriel SE, Michaud K. Epidemiological studies in incidence, prevalence, mortality, and comorbidity of the rheumatic diseases. Arthritis Research & Therapy. 2009;**11**(3):229

[77] Slater M, Perruccio AV, Badley EM. Musculoskeletal comorbidities in cardiovascular disease, diabetes and respiratory disease: The impact on activity limitations; a representative population-based study. BMC Public Health. 2011;**11**:77

[78] Radner H, Yoshida K, Frits M, Iannaccone C, Shadick NA, Weinblatt M, et al. The impact of multimorbidity status on treatment response in rheumatoid arthritis patients initiating disease-modifying anti-rheumatic drugs. Rheumatology. 2015;**54**(11):2076-2084

[79] Gunn JM, Ayton DR, Densley K, Pallant JF, Chondros P, Herrman HE, et al. The association between chronic illness, multimorbidity and depressive symptoms in an Australian primary care cohort. Social Psychiatry and Psychiatric Epidemiology. 2012;**47**(2):175-184

[80] Glynn LG, Valderas JM, Healy P, Burke E, Newell J, Gillespie P, et al. The prevalence of multimorbidity in primary care and its effect on health care utilization and cost. Family Practice. 2011;**28**(5):516-523

[81] Dominick CH, Blyth FM, Nicholas MK. Unpacking the burden: Understanding the relationships between chronic pain and comorbidity in the general population. Pain. 2012;**153**(2):293-304

[82] Higashi T, Wenger NS, Adams JL, Fung C, Roland M, McGlynn EA, et al. Relationship between number of medical conditions and quality of care. The New England Journal of Medicine. 2007;**356**(24):2496-2504

[83] Pham HH, Schrag D, O'Malley AS, Wu B, Bach PB. Care patterns in medicare and their implications for pay for performance. The New England Journal of Medicine. 2007;**356**(11):1130-1139

[84] Sav A, King MA, Whitty JA, Kendall E, McMillan SS, Kelly F, et al. Burden of treatment for chronic illness: A concept analysis and review of the literature. Health Expectations. 2015;**18**(3):312-324

[85] Solomon DH, Bitton A, Katz JN, Radner H, Brown EM, Fraenkel L. Review: Treat to target in rheumatoid arthritis: Fact, fiction, or hypothesis? Arthritis & Rhematology. 2014;**66**(4):775-782

[86] Farmer C, Fenu E, O'Flynn N, Guthrie B. Clinical assessment and management of multimorbidity: Summary of NICE guidance. BMJ. 2016;**354**:i4843

[87] Kernick D, Chew-Graham CA, O'Flynn N. Clinical assessment and management of multimorbidity: NICE guideline. The British Journal of General Practice. 2017;**67**(658):235-236

[88] Mead N, Bower P. Patient-centred consultations and outcomes in primary care: A review of the literature. Patient Education and Counseling. 2002;**48**(1):51-61

[89] Boyd CM, Fortin M. Future of multimorbidity research: How should understanding of multimorbidity inform health system design? Public Health Reviews. 2010;**32**(2):451-474

[90] Struckmann V, Leijten FRM, van Ginneken E, Kraus M, Reiss M, Spranger A, et al. Relevant models and elements of integrated care for multi-morbidity: Results of a scoping review. Health Policy. 2018;**122**(1):23-35

[91] Leijten FRM, Struckmann V, van Ginneken E, Czypionka T, Kraus M, Reiss M, et al. The SELFIE framework for integrated care for multi-morbidity: Development and description. Health Policy. 2018;**122**(1):12-22

[92] Hopman P, de Bruin SR, Forjaz MJ, Rodriguez-Blazquez C, Tonnara G, Lemmens LC, et al. Effectiveness of comprehensive care programs for patients with multiple chronic conditions or frailty: A systematic literature review. Health Policy. 2016;**120**(7):818-832

[93] Woolf AD. What healthcare services do people with musculoskeletal

conditions need? The role of rheumatology. Annals of the Rheumatic Diseases. 2007;**66**(3):281-282

[94] Dawes M. Co-morbidity: We need a guideline for each patient not a guideline for each disease. Family Practice. 2010;**27**(1):1-2

[95] Centers for Disease Control and Prevention's Arthritis Programme. 2016. Available from: https://www.cdc.gov/arthritis/data_statistics/disabilities-limitations.htm

[96] Lowe D, Taylor M, Hill S. Changing definitions altered multimorbidity prevalence, but not burden associations, in a musculoskeletal population. Journal of Clinical Epidemiology. 2016;**78**:116-126

[97] Woolf AD, Zeidler H, Haglund U, Carr AJ, Chaussade S, Cucinotta D, et al. Musculoskeletal pain in Europe: Its impact and a comparison of population and medical perceptions of treatment in eight European countries. Annals of the Rheumatic Diseases. 2004;**63**(4):342-347

Chapter 3

Cognitive Impairment in Chronic Lung Diseases

Emanuela Tudorache, Monica Marc, Daniel Traila and Diana Manolescu

Abstract

The increase in life expectancy has been accompanied by an escalation of age-related disease incidence. Mild cognitive impairment (MCI) is a decline of cognitive function higher than expected for a certain age, but not severe enough to meet the criteria for dementia. Hypoxemia, smoking history, ageing and several comorbidities are risk factors for both chronic respiratory diseases and cognitive deficit. Up to 70% of patients with chronic obstructive pulmonary disease (COPD), obstructive sleep apnea (OSA) or idiopathic pulmonary fibrosis (IPF) have a form of cognitive impairment. Furthermore, a low neuropsychological performance is an independent predictor of disability and mortality in these populations. Efficient tools for cognitive assessment have been validated for these patients and should be used for better clinical outcomes. The physiopathological mechanisms, clinical impact and prevention strategies for cognitive dysfunction in chronic respiratory diseases will be detailed in the following chapter.

Keywords: cognitive dysfunction, hypoxemia, chronic obstructive pulmonary disease, obstructive sleep apnea, idiopathic pulmonary fibrosis

1. Introduction

In the era of antibiotics, vaccines and other medical innovations, life expectancy has increased worldwide, which has led to an enhanced prevalence chronic diseases. Only in the USA, the Department of Health and Human Services estimates that by the year 2040, 82.3 million Americans (21.7% of the population) will be over 65 years of age [1]. Consequently, age-related illnesses that cause a significant morbidity and mortality will become a rising public health problem. At the same time, there is an increase in the prevalence of multimorbidity, defined by the coexistence of two or more chronic pathologies in the same individual. Studies show that in individuals that are over 60 years old, the multimorbidity range is from 55 to 98% [2]. Multimorbidity is associated with functional decline, disability, poor quality of life, higher emergency care and hospitalizations rates, polypharmacy and increased healthcare costs, all of which are a great burden for society [3].

The concept of cognitive impairment has been carefully analysed in the last two decades, given the devastating consequences of this problem, mainly among elderly populations. Cognitive function can be divided into six large domains: language (verbal fluency and comprehension), learning ability and memory (work memory and memory-based tagging), attention, executive functions (planning and problem solving), praxis (motor-ideative, ideative and visual constructive) and visuospatial function [4].

Mild cognitive impairment (MCI) is defined as a cognitive dysfunction more severe than normal age-related cognitive decline or education level, but not severe enough to significantly interfere with daily function [5]. MCI exceeds the "age-related" decline in cognition healthy individuals experience but does not meet the criteria for dementia. Furthermore, not all cases of MCI will progress towards dementia.

In the general population, studies have shown a prevalence of MCI between 10 and 20% in older adults [5]. However, cognitive impairment is heavily underdiagnosed and undertreated by primary care physicians. There are several screening tools that can identify those with a high risk of MCI such as the Mini-Mental State Examination (MMSE), Montreal Cognitive Assessment (MoCA), Saint Louis University Mental Status Examination (SLUMS) or Rapid Cognitive Screen. Once the diagnosis of cognitive dysfunction is determined, it is essential to establish the aetiology and the contributing factors and to evaluate if there are any reversible causes. Every practitioner should be familiar with these questionnaires, especially MMSE, and should use them whenever they suspect a person of MCI.

Neuroanatomical structures and their function can be assessed by neuroimaging techniques. Computed tomography (CT) scan and magnetic resonance imaging (MRI) can analyse the brain structure and exclude conditions such as strokes, brain tumours or vascular malformation. The fluorodeoxyglucose positron-emission tomography (FDG-PET) scan, mostly used for research purposes, can evaluate the brain function and seems to be more sensitive than MRI in MCI diagnosis. This tool uses a radioactive glucose tracer which binds to highly active brain areas. The presence of hypometabolic areas in the temporal or parietal lobe is a sign of neurodegeneration. Subjects who develop these hypometabolic areas have a higher risk of progression from MCI to dementia [6, 7]. For research purposes, there are several biomarkers used for the diagnosis of MCI and dementia, but the lack of standardization regarding optimal cutoff points limits their clinical utility [8].

There are well-established risk factors for developing MCI: age, male gender, family history of cognitive impairment, the presence of the apolipoprotein E allele, smoking and low educational level [9]. Moreover, one study, which aimed to determine if multimorbidity could be a risk factor for mild cognitive impairment and dementia, found that individuals who associate at least two of the following, hypertension, hyperlipidemia, coronary artery disease and arthritis, had a very high risk of MCI [3].

Recent studies showed that some chronic respiratory conditions, such as chronic obstructive pulmonary disease (COPD), obstructive sleep apnea (OSA) or idiopathic pulmonary fibrosis (IPF), have an important impact on cognitive function. There are discrepancies regarding the reported prevalence of cognitive dysfunction among the conditions listed above, which can be explained by study design and limitations: diagnostic methods for cognitive impairment (psychometric tools or neuroimaging), small sample size or inappropriate control group, assessment moment (stable phase/exacerbation), the severity of the airflow limitation, presence of hypoxia and the use of long-term oxygen therapy. Multiple confounders can also contribute to the large variation of data regarding prevalence: age, education level, smoking history, comorbidities, etc.

2. Cognitive impairment in obstructive sleep apnea

Sleep apnea syndrome is a disorder of breathing during sleep, characterized by total or partial obstruction of the upper airways leading to hypoxia and hypercapnia, plus increased respiratory effort [10]. These features produce micro-awakenings that result in disruption of sleep and changes in neuronal activity. All of these are potential mechanisms for cognitive deficiency [11].

In adults, the prevalence of OSA increases significantly with age. Between 30 and 49 years, 10% of men and 3% of women are diagnosed, increasing to 17 and 9%, respectively, for 50–70 years [12] and with increasing prevalence among postmenopausal women [13]. These percentages are higher than those published 10 years ago, due to the fact that obesity is increasing among the population of developing countries [14]. More worryingly, the true prevalence may be underestimated as many people with OSA remain undiagnosed.

Nighttime symptoms are noisy snoring, non-restful sleep, nocturia, sweating and dry mouth. One of the most common daytime symptoms in patients with OSA is daytime sleepiness. This greatly influences the quality of life and cognitive performance.

OSA has been associated with a wide range of psychological problems such as depression, anxiety, neurocognitive dysfunction, especially attention, alertness, memory and learning, phenomena due to fragmentation of sleep and intermittent hypoxemia [15–17]. Fragmentation of sleep, sleep deprivation and the association of excessive daytime sleepiness are proposed mechanisms that underlie cognitive impairment through their impact on attention [18, 19].

The exact prevalence of cognitive disorders and their severity due to multiple comorbidities with which this syndrome is associated is not known in adult patients with OSA.

2.1 Risk factors for cognitive deficits in OSA patients

There are numerous OSA comorbidities that can influence cognitive function, such as treatment-resistant hypertension [20], diabetes [21], COPD, congestive heart failure, strokes [22], smoking [23] and alcoholism [24]. Also age, sex (male), obesity and the use of psychoactive drugs are considered independent risk factors [25].

Ageing itself causes decline in cognitive function, and the presence of OSA in these patients leads to further brain injury, with cognitive impairment being more obvious [26]. It is also known that smoking, through its damaging effects on blood vessels and circulation, increases the risk of dementia, both vascular and Alzheimer's, as well as neurocognitive decline not associated with dementia [27].

Another important factor in the association of OSA with cognitive decline is, it seems, the genetic factor. Thus, studies show that the presence of apolipoprotein E4 (ApoE4) is associated with an increased incidence of cognitive disorders [28].

High blood pressure is associated with cognitive decline, both when isolated and in the presence of metabolic syndrome, especially due to the presence of cardiovascular risk factors [29].

Also, the presence of hypothyroidism in patients with OSA may accelerate cognitive decline, and current data are not sufficient to demonstrate whether the treatment ameliorates the decline phenomena [30].

Moderate alcohol consumption may protect against dementia, but significant alcohol consumption is associated with cognitive impairment, which is manifested by loss of memory, impaired personality and impaired judgement [24]. Alcohol intake before bedtime affects sleep architecture [31]. In addition, depending on the quantity, the instability of the upper airways may increase [32]. Thus, excessive alcohol use by patients with OSA may lead to more severe cognitive deficits.

Another common comorbidity of OSA is stroke, which, independently, is accompanied by a cognitive deficiency and even dementia. Studies show that up to 30% of patients with stroke can develop dementia [33, 34]. And psychoactive medication, e.g. benzodiazepines, narcotics and barbiturates, can aggravate OSA and increase attention and alertness problems [35, 36].

Studies carried out over time have shown structural and functional changes in the brain, resulting in cognitive deficiency. There are studies that, by MRI techniques, have shown decrease of grey matter in the hippocampus; cerebellum; frontal, parietal and temporal lobes; as well as the anterior cingulate cortex [37–39]. Also, a decrease in the hippocampus was observed, which plays an important role in memory consolidation. The white matter changes reported by O'Donoghue et al. indicate that axonal or glial pathology is also present in OSA, consistent with other previous findings [40].

2.2 Physiopathology of cognitive impairment in patients with OSA

Studies on the cardiovascular effects of OSA have shown that the disorder results in changes in vascular structure and function, these changes being frequently encountered in other hypoxic populations [41]. It is assumed that hypoxia would have a direct effect on the neuropsychic in patients with OSA, with existing similar mechanisms in terms of cardiovascular changes and brain vessels. Hypoxia produces immediate vasodilation, being a protective mechanism to more efficiently distribute oxygen to the affected organ. Studies have shown that this protective mechanism does not exist in patients with OSA [42]. One potential reason why these patients do not have a response to hypoxemia is because they suffer from repeated episodes of hypoxemia (over five events/h) and desaturation, not just a sustained hypoxic event. Thus, the post-episode recovery time being limited, it is not possible to estimate whether there is a protective response to recurrent hypoxic events, but it is assumed that the vessels would suffer [43].

Therefore, in patients with OSA, there are lesions due to hypoxia and reperfusion with increased lipid peroxidation. This process involves the oxidation of polyunsaturated fatty acids with the formation of reactive oxygen species and toxic products, having potential damaging effects for the brain and heart.

Also, in patients with vascular pathology, endothelial dysfunction is present. In patients with OSA, imbalances between vasoconstrictive mediators (higher thromboxane and endothelin levels) and vasodilators (nitric oxide, prostacycline) appear, and nitric oxide production has been shown to decrease in OSA. This imbalance predisposes to atherosclerosis [44]. Thus, the effects on cerebral flow, as well as hypoxia, may cause the onset of cerebral infarctions, resulting in vascular dementia. The presence of endothelial dysfunction, with the onset of neurocognitive deficits, has been described even in studies performed in the paediatric population [16].

There are authors who consider that the cognitive impairment in OSA represents the short-term consequence of the poor quality of sleep manifested by daytime sleepiness or attention difficulties. Studies have shown specific and localized frontal lobe involvement, responsible for the executory dysfunction observed in OSA [45]. The basis of this hypothesis is that sleep disruption reduces the efficiency of restoration processes in the prefrontal cortex that will also lead to cellular and biochemical stress. These processes, in turn, disrupt functional homeostasis, altering the viability of neuronal and glial cells [46–48]. The severity of sleep fragmentation is associated with attention deficit and decreased alertness, and the overall cognitive deficit is the consequence of hypoxia. Due to sleep fragmentation, alteration of blood gases and changes of homeostasis in the frontal lobe and hippocampus leads to memory impairment and executory function deficiency.

2.3 The effects of CPAP therapy on cognitive deficiency

A direct consequence of OSA, with impact on both personal and social levels, is the loss of vigilance. This increases the risk of traffic accidents in untreated patients, which is why it is important to diagnose and treat this condition as early as possible [49]. Election treatment of OSA is continuous positive airway pressure (CPAP) therapy. This method was first described in 1981 [50]. Since then, technological progress has been made to suit the needs of patients. Also, in order to improve treatment adherence, device manufacturers have considered the importance of producing mask interfaces that match the user's physiognomy. This variety improves comfort and reduces air leakage. The use of CPAP for at least 4 h of sleep during a 24-h period defines a minimum acceptable level in terms of a beneficial therapeutic response. Thus, for maximum benefit, most clinicians recommend using the device for the entire duration of sleep [51].

Canessa et al. studied the effects of CPAP therapy on neurocognitive changes in 17 OSA patients. Therefore, voxel-based morphometry determinations showed significant post-therapy improvements in the cognition level, together with the increase of the volume of the grey matter in the frontal lobe and hippocampus [52]. This is why early diagnosis and initiation of CPAP therapy could prevent, in the medium and long term, the cognitive impairment. In summary, this study provides the first evidence that structural brain abnormalities exist in hypoxemia-sensitive regions and they may change with treatment. These results suggest that even the negative neurological effects of hypoxemia can be reversed with consistent and complete treatment. Therefore, adherence to CPAP treatment can lead not only to clinical recovery but also to structural brain recovery. It should be noted that the patients in this study showed a positive response to treatment. MRI may thus be used as a marker, to evaluate the response to treatment [53].

There are studies that show that use of CPAP over 12 months also leads to significant recovery of the impaired white matter, including corpus callosum, with important impact on improving cognition [54]. There are also numerous studies evaluating the effects of CPAP therapy in stroke patients who develop OSA. The stroke can aggravate functional changes and cognition. A study conducted in Korea highlights the beneficial effects of the therapy and suggests that this treatment should be considered as part of the rehabilitation programme for stroke patients. Thereby, CPAP therapy applied to patients with subacute stroke for a relatively short period of time leads to an improvement in sleep quality, daytime sleepiness and cognitive function. Further research regarding the improvement of neurological and functional status among stroke patients, who have received long-term CPAP treatment, is needed [55].

In conclusion, although there are numerous studies that have focused on the association of OSA with cognitive deficits, things are far from fully elucidated. Variate and numerous comorbidities, including ageing, hypoxemia, genetic factors, strokes, etc., independently influence these deficits. Untreated OSA is correlated with changes in brain structure and function through cell death, grey matter destruction, inflammatory changes and decreased white matter integrity. Unlike other pathologies, however, initiating CPAP therapy as early as possible prevents the installation of the cognitive deficiency or improves it if it is already installed.

3. Cognitive impairment in chronic obstructive pulmonary disease

COPD is a common disease, characterized by persistent respiratory symptoms and airflow limitation caused by significant exposure to noxious particles and gases.

COPD is an important cause of morbidity and premature death. According to the WHO, by 2030 it will be the third cause of death worldwide [56].

A large meta-analysis which included 23,116 patients with COPD showed an alarming prevalence of MCI, up to 32%, compared with the prevalence of 10–20% in the general population [57]. Furthermore, in time this mild cognitive decline seems to aggravate, and these patients will have an increased risk to develop multi-infarct dementia or Alzheimer's disease [58].

3.1 Risk factors for cognitive impairment in patients with COPD

The origin of the cognitive impairment COPD patients is still not well established. Several pathological relays can interfere: smoking, ageing, severe lung disease, hypoxemia, hypercapnia, systemic inflammation, oxidative stress, endothelial dysfunction, comorbidities, sedentary lifestyle and genetic factors.

3.2 Physiopathology of cognitive impairment in patients with COPD

From all the above, hypoxemia seems to be the most important risk factor. Not only continuous hypoxemia but also the intermittent one (during efforts, sleep and daily activities) can cause brain damage [59]. Moreover, a study showed that during COPD exacerbations when hypoxemia worsens, patients have significantly altered cognitive scores compared with those recorded in stable phases and age-matched controls [60]. Neurologic impairment also worsens with COPD progression. In the severe pulmonary disease, altered MMSE scores were reported in 64% of cases [61]. The most common abnormalities in the MMSE included construction (39%), attention (31%), verbal recall (26%), visuospatial orientation (24%) and language (13%). In tasks that required drawing (e.g. an analogue clock with a set time) or other tasks that required judgement, poor performance was associated with a higher mortality [62]. In addition, Chang et al. in a 3-year prospective study showed that the association between COPD and cognitive dysfunction led to increased disability, hospital rate and mortality [63].

One of the most elaborate studies was performed by Dodd et al. [4] who focused on non-hypoxemic COPD patients and combined different brain function assessment techniques such as magnetic resonance diffusion tensor imaging, resting state functional MRI and neuropsychological questionnaires. The report showed that these individuals had decreased integrity of the white matter, dysfunction of grey matter and poor performance in the cognitive questionnaires, compared with age-matched controls. The most significant deficits recorded through imaging techniques were poor executive function, low processing speed and episodic and working memory impairment, which all corresponded with the deficits seen on the MMSE test.

The Rotterdam Study used high-resolution MRI to evaluate cerebral structures in subjects with COPD and reported a higher frequency of cerebral microbleeds. This observation supports the concept of cerebral small-vessel disease that leads to cognitive decline via cerebral micro-bleeding areas. They also increased the MRI performance by introducing voxel-based morphometry analysis. Through this technique, they demonstrated for the first time that even stable COPD patients, who had subclinical cognitive impairment, presented grey matter volume alterations on MRI [64].

Other MRI studies revealed a significantly loss of grey matter in numerous brain areas: precuneus, right inferior parietal lobule, right superior temporal gyrus/middle temporal gyrus, hippocampus, limbic and paralimbic structures, cingulate, amygdala, etc. The common aspect in these studies is heterogeneity and broad distribution of the lesions which could explain the multiple and variate neurologic manifestations these patients experience. Moreover, neuroimaging showed that parietal lobule and precuneus are also altered in Alzheimer's disease.

The psychometric profile impairment correlates with variable components of COPD such as disease severity, exacerbations, hypoxemia or hypercapnia [58]. For accurate results it is indicated to use a battery of tests, not a single one. The most commonly affected cognitive domains are memory, attention, motor and executive function, naming ability and visuospatial orientation [65].

On the other hand, COPD cases without comorbidities are rare. This disease is frequently associated with both respiratory pathologies, like pulmonary hypertension (3–84%), obstructive sleep apnea (58–88%) or lung cancer (3–22%), and non-respiratory comorbidities such as systemic arterial hypertension (14–71%), ischemic heart disease (4–68%), depression (12–49%) and diabetes mellitus type 2 (10–33%) [66]. Although the number of comorbidities rises with age, special caution should be addressed to cognitive-related comorbidities: cerebrovascular diseases, cardiovascular pathology, diabetes mellitus and sleep apnea syndrome. These pathologies should be managed according to current guidelines.

3.3 The effects of therapy and pulmonary rehabilitation on cognitive deficiency in COPD patients

Studies show that 50% of COPD patients abandon the prescribed inhaled medication and the oxygen therapy during the first year of therapy and just 25% use oxygen therapy for activities outside their house [67]. Moreover, older COPD patients and those with cognitive impairment have even lower adherence levels to inhalation therapy. The cognitive status impacts patient's ability to recall when and how to use the inhaler devices. Poor executive functioning is often associated with a "knowing–doing" discrepancy [68]. All these factors listed above have a negative impact on treatment adherence and self-management.

The dyspnea–inactivity–muscular dysfunction circle developed by COPD patients will lead to isolation, depression and low adherence to pulmonary rehabilitation programmes. Given the multifactorial aspects of adherence and the high prevalence of MCI among COPD population, pulmonary rehabilitation programmes should be tailored to subject's needs.

On the other hand, these programmes have a positive feedback on respiratory symptoms and neurologic function. Therefore, screening for these comorbidities should be considered during baseline pulmonary rehabilitation assessment [69]. Cognitive behavioural therapy or psychological support should be considered when psychological difficulties interfere with disease self-management and adherence [67].

Another condition that should not be ignored in patients with COPD is gait impairment. More evidence suggests that muscle loss, reduced exercise capacity and functional mobility is leading to an important risk of falls. Interventions that include coordination, balance and strength training proved to be effective in older adults [70]. However, balance training and fall prevention strategies are still not mentioned by the pulmonary rehabilitation guidelines, and very few rehabilitation centres have a standardized balance assessment.

Although regular use of long-term oxygen therapy (LTOT) is correlated with a reduced risk of cognitive impairment in subjects with COPD, it is still under debate when and to whom it should be addressed. However, in patients who develop intermittent hypoxemia (during effort or sleep), earlier oxygen supplementation should be considered in order to prevent irreversible neurologic damage [56].

During COPD exacerbations in hypercapnic respiratory failure, non-invasive ventilation is a key management tool which markedly reduces mortality and morbidity. Prompt initiation of CPAP therapy prevents the installation of the cognitive impairment [71].

4. Cognitive impairment in idiopathic pulmonary fibrosis

Pulmonary fibrosis describes the group of fibrosing interstitial lung diseases (ILDs) that causes progressive scarring of the alveolar interstitium, often leading to hypoxemic respiratory failure. ILDs encompass a large and varied group of parenchymal lung disorders, including diseases of unknown cause (idiopathic interstitial pneumonias), as well as those associated with other diseases (connective tissue disease-associated ILDs, chronic sarcoidosis) or environmental exposures (chronic hypersensitivity pneumonitis).

Idiopathic pulmonary fibrosis (IPF), the most extensively studied type of ILD, is a relentlessly progressive lung disease with a prognosis that can be worse than many cancers. With a median survival time of 2.5–3.5 years after diagnosis [72], IPF portends substantial morbidity and mortality outcomes, not all of which are directly related to the progressive fibrotic disease itself.

This older population with a median age of 66 years at diagnosis frequently experience various comorbidities, which influence the clinical spectrum, progression and mortality of the disease. An analysis of 272 IPF patients reported that 58% of cases had one, two or three comorbid conditions, 30% had four to seven comorbid conditions and only 12% had no comorbidities [73]. Respiratory comorbidities, including emphysema (8–34%), obstructive sleep apnea (58–88%), lung cancer (3–22%) and pulmonary hypertension (3–84%), were common in many studies, although estimates vary widely depending on the source population. Non-respiratory comorbidities such as gastro-oesophageal reflux (30–80%), systemic arterial hypertension (14–71%), ischaemic heart disease (4–68%), diabetes mellitus type 2 (10–33%) and depression (12–49%) are also highly prevalent [74, 75].

4.1 Risk factors for cognitive deficits in patients with IPF

Related to IPF or associated morbidity, there are several potential factors and conditions for the emergence of a cognitive deficit. Hypoxemia, a history of smoking, ageing and chronic evolution of the disease are potential elements for the emergence of a cognitive deficit.

Difficulties in breathing (increased intrinsic elastic load of respiratory muscles and stimulation of peripheral mechanoreceptors) [76], night cough, drugs, hypoxemia and obstructive apnea can all alter the quality of life.

4.2 Physiopathology of cognitive impairment in patients with IPF

IPF patients develop progressive ventilatory restriction and exercise intolerance. Alteration of blood gases is a common feature in IPF pathophysiology. Patients experience transient or continuous hypoxia resulting in a substantial cumulative time with an SpO_2 below 90%. Nocturnal hypoxia is common in chronic fibrotic interstitial lung diseases, both in patients who associate OSA, as those without this comorbidity. In the absence of OSA, nocturnal hypoxia could be a result of alveolar hypoventilation, altered ventilation-perfusion ratio and a desaturation trend, due to patients on the abrupt portion of the oxygen-haemoglobin dissociation curve [77, 78].

Epidemiologic research has shown that besides genetic and environmental factors, such as lifestyles and cardiovascular risk factors, decreased lung function is also associated with dementia and cognitive impairment in the general population.

In a large population-based cohort enrolled in the Atherosclerosis Risk in Communities Study [79], the presence of a restrictive ventilatory pattern was associated with worse performance in cognitive assessments and with an increased risk of dementia hospitalization.

A recent prospective study [80] found that patients with restrictive lung disease have almost twice the chance of developing dementia or mild cognitive impairment as healthy individuals. Researchers followed more than 14.000 middle-aged people for over 23 years. Lung disease and impaired lung function were associated with greater risk of dementia and mild cognitive impairment through both Alzheimer's disease and cerebrovascular aetiologies. Although both COPD and restrictive impairment were associated with increased risk of the dementia phenotypes, magnitudes of association were most pronounced for restrictive impairment. There were no differences between smokers and non-smokers.

Different pathogenic mechanisms could explain the association of lung function with cognitive performance and risk of dementia. Chronic hypoxia might lead to ischaemic brain injury and neurodegeneration as prospective studies have found that individuals with low lung function or reduced arterial oxygen saturation are more likely to develop white matter lesions and lacunar infarcts [81, 82].

A restrictive ventilatory pattern has been associated with the incidence of diabetes and subclinical atherosclerosis and an increased risk of cardiovascular outcomes [83, 84]. In turn, diabetes and cardiovascular disease might cause cognitive impairment and increase the risk of dementia.

Worse lung function might cause cognitive impairment and dementia through the development of a pro-inflammatory state. High levels of C-reactive protein, elevated in individuals with reduced lung function, have been associated with a higher risk of dementia [85, 86].

In IPF, a disease with a potential rapid and frequent development of hypoxemia, it is surprising that cognitive impairment has been investigated in very few studies.

In a limited study [87], with only seven IPF patients undergoing pulmonary rehabilitation, applying a battery of five psychometric tests (recall of verbal information, sustained visual attention, efficiency in completing sequential tasks, verbal fluency, visuospatial and graphomotor proficiency) found impaired cognition only on the level of visual attention.

A prospective, observational study examining cognitive function in 30 IPF patients with normal oxygen saturations and comparing them to COPD and smoking controls demonstrated that almost half of IPF patients have mild cognitive dysfunction, unexplained by age [88].

In a prospective, cross-sectional, descriptive study [89], Bors et al. showed that individuals with severe IPF have worse cognitive function than those with mild-to-moderate disease and controls. Participants were evaluated through five neuropsychological tests that assessed various domains of cognitive function: speed for attention, sequencing, mental flexibility, visual search and motor function, information processing speed, selective attention, cognitive flexibility, executive function, assessment of verbal recall and recognition and specific cognitive deficits related to accessibility of lexical and semantic information. Severe IPF patients had a significantly inferior performance on tasks requiring speed-divided attention and slower processing speeds when requiring suppression of a familiar response. They are also more likely to have poorer health-related quality of life and symptoms of depression.

A cross-sectional study aimed to assess cognition in IPF and to identify clinical cognition modifiers, and 23 IPF patients were evaluated using the Montreal Cognitive Assessment (MoCA) [66]. As it has been previously mentioned, MoCA is a screening instrument with high specificity and sensitivity for detecting early cognitive impairments and is validated in multiple settings and disorders. MoCA evaluates several cognitive domains (short-term memory, visuospatial abilities, executive functioning, attention, concentration and working memory, language, orientation to time and place) to differentiate healthy cognitive ageing from mild cognitive impairment [90]. The study found a mild cognitive impairment in patients with IPF that is related to the areas of visuospatial abilities, language and working memory. Obstructive sleep apnea was highly prevalent in these patients (more than 80% of cases), and there was a significant correlation between cognitive function and the severity of apnea hypopnea index. Poor sleep quality is frequently met in IPF through sleep breathing disorders, including OSA, implying increased sleep fragmentation, decreased slow wave and REM sleep, as well as sleep oxygen desaturation [91].

4.3 Management of cognitive deficiency in IPF patients

Health-related quality of life is especially important in this patient population, given the lack of treatment options, poor mortality and rapid progression of the disease. The morbidity associated with IPF has a wide and profound impact on the patient's quality of life. Therefore, cognition level and other patient-centred outcomes are important goals to be evaluated in clinical research and practice. For IPF we do not currently have a specific cognitive assessment tool, so researchers have used validated tools in cognition analysis of other chronic respiratory diseases. The potential problem is that these tools cannot capture many of the effects of IPF on patients' lives.

5. Conclusion

Patients with chronic respiratory conditions, such as obstructive sleep apnea, chronic obstructive pulmonary disease or idiopathic pulmonary fibrosis, commonly associate cognitive impairment. Neurologic assessment should be included in the routine diagnostic algorithm of these conditions, in order to appreciate the overall impact of the disease, on patient's quality of life and prognosis. Physicians who notice signs of memory loss, disorientation, gait impairment or even poor adherence to pharmacologic/nonpharmacologic treatment, should screen their patients for cognitive dysfunction. For a better outcome, subjects who are identified with mild cognitive impairment by a screening tool should be referred for a thorough evaluation to a neurologist, and the chronic lung disease management should be tailored according to individual's needs.

Author details

Emanuela Tudorache[1]*, Monica Marc[1], Daniel Traila[1] and Diana Manolescu[2]

1 Department of Pulmonology, "Victor Babes" University of Medicine and Pharmacy, Timişoara, Romania

2 Department of Radiology, "Victor Babes" University of Medicine and Pharmacy, Timişoara, Romania

*Address all correspondence to: tudorache_emanuela@yahoo.com

References

[1] http://www.acl.gov/sites/default/files/about-acl/2017-03/FY15OAAReportCongress_2017-1-24.docx

[2] Marengoni A, Roso-Llorach A, Vetrano DL, et al. Patterns of multimorbidity in a population-based cohort of older people: Sociodemographic, lifestyle, clinical, and functional differences. The Journals of Gerontology Series A Biological Sciences. 9 March 2020;**75**(4):798-805. DOI: 10.1093/gerona/glz137

[3] Vassilaki M, Aakre JA, Cha RH, et al. Multimorbidity and risk of mild cognitive impairment. Journal of the American Geriatrics Society. 2015;**63**(9):1783-1790

[4] Dodd JW, Chung AW, van den Broek MD, et al. Brain structure and function in chronic obstructive pulmonary disease: A multimodal cranial magnetic resonance imaging study. American Journal of Respiratory and Critical Care Medicine. 2012;**186**(3):240-245

[5] American Psychiatric Association. Diagnostic and Statistical Manual of Mental Disorders. 5th ed. Arlington, VA: American Psychiatric Association; 2013

[6] Yuan Y, Gu ZX, Wei WS. Fluorodeoxyglucose-positron-emission tomography, single-photon emission tomography, and structural MR imaging for prediction of rapid conversion to Alzheimer disease in patients with mild cognitive impairment: A meta-analysis. AJNR. American Journal of Neuroradiology. 2009;**30**:404-410

[7] Karow DS, McEvoy LK, Fennema-Notestine C, et al. Relative capability of MR imaging and FDG PET to depict changes associated with prodromal and early Alzheimer disease. Radiology. 2010;**256**:932-942

[8] Sanford AM. Mild cognitive impairment. Clinics in Geriatric Medicine. 2017;**33**(3):325-337

[9] Ng TP, Feng L, Nyunt MS, et al. Metabolic syndrome and the risk of mild cognitive impairment and progression to dementia: Follow-up of the Singapore Longitudinal Ageing Study Cohort. JAMA Neurology. 2016;**73**(4):456-463

[10] Edwards BA, Eckert DJ, Jordan AS. Obstructive sleep apnoea pathogenesis from mild to severe: Is it all the same? Respirology. 2016;**22**:33-42

[11] EEG arousals: Scoring rules and examples. A preliminary report from the Sleep Disorders Atlas Task Force of the American Sleep Disorders Association. Sleep. 1992;**15**:173-184

[12] Peppard PE, Young T, Barnet JH, et al. Increased prevalence of sleep disordered breathing in adults. American Journal of Epidemiology. 2013;**117**:1006-1014

[13] Kapsimalis F, Kryger M. Sleep breathing disorders in the U.S. female population. Journal of Women's Health (Larchmt). 2009;**18**:1211-1219

[14] Senaratna CV, Perret JL, Lodge CJ, et al. Prevalence of obstructive sleep apnea in the general population: A systematic review. Sleep Medicine Reviews. 2017;**34**:70-81

[15] Salorio CF, White DA, Piccirillo J, et al. Learning, memory, and executive control in individuals with obstructive sleep apnea syndrome. Journal of Clinical and Experimental Neuropsychology. 2002;**24**(1):93-100

[16] Beebe DW, Gozal D. Obstructive sleep apnea and the prefrontal cortex: Towards a comprehensive model linking nocturnal upper airway obstruction to daytime cognitive and behavioral deficits. Journal of Sleep Research. 2002;**11**(1):1-16

[17] Sutton AM. Executive functioning in the presence of sleep disordered breathing. Dissertation Abstracts International: Section B: The Sciences and Engineering. 2008;**69**(1-B):701

[18] Verstraeten E, Cluydts R. Executive control of attention in sleep apnea patients: Theoretical concepts and methodological considerations. Sleep Medicine Reviews. 2004;**8**(4):257-267

[19] Verstraeten E, Cluydts R, Pevernagie D, et al. Executive function in sleep apnea: Controlling for attentional capacity in assessing executive attention. Sleep. 2004;**27**(4):685-693

[20] Logan AG, Perlikowski SM, Mente A, et al. High prevalence of unrecognized sleep apnoea in drug-resistant hypertension. Journal of Hypertension. 2001;**19**(12):2271-2277

[21] Elmasry A, Lindberg E, Berne C, et al. Sleep-disordered breathing and glucose metabolism in hypertensive men: A population-based study. Journal of Internal Medicine. 2001;**249**(2):153-161

[22] Parra O, Arboix A, Bechich S, et al. Time course of sleep related breathing disorders in first-ever stroke or transient ischemic attack. American Journal of Respiratory and Critical Care Medicine. 2000;**161**(2 pt 1):375-380

[23] Wetter DW, Young TB, Bidwell TR, et al. Smoking as a risk factor for sleep-disordered breathing. Archives of Internal Medicine. 1994;**154**(19):2219-2224

[24] Chan KK, Chiu KC, Chu LW. Association between alcohol consumption and cognitive impairment in Southern Chinese older adults. International Journal of Geriatric Psychiatry. 2010;**25**(12):1272-1279

[25] Lal C, Strange C, Bachman D. Neurocognitive impairment in obstructive sleep apnea. Chest. 2012;**141**(6):1601-1610

[26] Petersen RC, Roberts RO, Knopman DS, et al. The Mayo Clinic Study of Aging . Prevalence of mild cognitive impairment is higher in men. Neurology. 2010;**75**(10):889-897

[27] Bekris LM, Yu CE, Bird TD, et al. Genetics of Alzheimer disease. Journal of Geriatric Psychiatry and Neurology. 2010;**23**(4):213-227

[28] Kadotani H, Kadotani T, Young T, et al. Association between apolipoprotein E epsilon4 and sleep-disordered breathing in adults. The Journal of the American Medical Association. 2001;**285**(22):2888-2890

[29] Panza F, Frisardi V, Capurso C, et al. Metabolic syndrome and cognitive impairment: Current epidemiology and possible underlying mechanisms. Journal of Alzheimer's Disease. 2010;**21**(3):691-724

[30] Lin CC, Tsan KW, Chen PJ. The relationship between sleep apnea syndrome and hypothyroidism. Chest. 1992;**102**(6):1663-1667

[31] Feige B, Gann H, Brueck R, et al. Effects of alcohol on polysomnographically recorded sleep in healthy subjects. Alcoholism, Clinical and Experimental Research. 2006;**30**(9):1527-1537

[32] Issa FG, Sullivan CE. Upper airway closing pressures in snorers. Journal of Applied Physiology. 1984;**57**(2):528-535

[33] Minoguchi K, Yokoe T, Tazaki T, et al. Silent brain infarction and platelet activation in obstructive sleep apnea. American Journal of Respiratory and Critical Care Medicine. 2007;**175**(6):612-617

[34] Tatemichi TK, Foulkes MA, Mohr JP, et al. Dementia in stroke survivors in the Stroke Data Bank cohort. Prevalence, incidence, risk factors, and computed tomographic fi ndings. Stroke. 1990;**21**(6):858-866

[35] Moore AR, O'Keeffe ST. Drug-induced cognitive impairment in the elderly. Drugs & Aging. 1999;**15**(1):15-28

[36] Shirani A, Paradiso S, Dyken ME. The impact of atypical antipsychotic use on obstructive sleep apnea: A pilot study and literature review. Sleep Medicine. 2011;**12**(6):591-597

[37] Gale SD, Hopkins RO. Effects of hypoxia on the brain: Neuroimaging and neuropsychological findings following carbon monoxide poisoning and obstructive sleep apnea. Journal of the International Neuropsychological Society. 2004;**10**(1):60-71

[38] Macey PM, Henderson LA, Macey KE, et al. Brain morphology associated with obstructive sleep apnea. American Journal of Respiratory and Critical Care Medicine. 2002;**166**(10):1382-1387

[39] Morrell MJ, McRobbie DW, Quest RA, et al. Changes in brain morphology associated with obstructive sleep apnea. Sleep Medicine. 2003;**4**(5):451-454

[40] O'Donoghue FJ, Wellard RM, Rochford PD, et al. Magnetic resonance spectroscopy and neurocognitive dysfunction in obstructive sleep apnea before and after CPAP treatment. Sleep. 2012;**35**:41-48

[41] Parkinson J, Dalley J, Cardinal R, et al. Nucleus accumbens dopamine depletion impairs both acquisition and performance of appetitive Pavlovian approach behaviour: Implications for mesoaccumbens dopamine function. Behavioural Brain Research. 2002;**137**(1-2):149-163

[42] Kato M, Roberts-Thomson P, Phillips BG, et al. Impairment of endothelium dependent vasodilation of resistance vessels in patients with obstructive sleep apnea. 2000;**102**(21):2607-2610

[43] Aloia MS, Ardet JT, Davis JD, et al. Neuropsychological sequelae of obstructive sleep apnea-hypopnea syndrome: A critical review. Journal of the International Neuropsychological Society. 2004;**10**:772-785

[44] Nedeljkovic ZS, Gokce N, Loscalzo J. Mechanisms of oxidative stress and vascular dysfunction. Postgraduate Medical Journal. 2003;**79**(930):195-199

[45] Gozal D, Kheirandish-Gozal L, Bhattacharjee R, et al. Neurocognitive and endothelial dysfunction in children with obstructive sleep apnea. Pediatrics. 2010;**126**(5):e1161-e1167

[46] Horne JA. Why We Sleep. Oxford: Oxford University Press; 1988

[47] Madsen PL. Blood flow and oxygen uptake in the human brain during various states of sleep and wakefulness. Acta Neurologica Scandinavica. 1993;**148**:S3-S27

[48] Maquet P. Sleep function (s) and cerebral metabolism. Behavioural Brain Research. 1995;**69**:75-83

[49] Findley LJ, Levinson MP, Bonnie RJ. Driving performance and automobile accidents in patients with sleep apnea. Clinics in Chest Medicine. 1992;**13**(3):427-435

[50] Sullivan CE, Issa FG, Berthon-Jones M, et al. Reversal of obstructive sleep apnoea by continuous positive airway pressure applied through the nares. Lancet. 1981;**1**(8225):862-865

[51] Antic NA, Catcheside P, Buchan C, et al. The effect of CPAP in normalizing daytime sleepiness, quality of life, and neurocognitive function in patients with moderate to severe OSA. Sleep. 2011;**34**(1):111-119

[52] Canessa N, Castronovo V, Cappa SF, et al. Obstructive sleep apnea: Brain structural changes and neurocognitive function before and after treatment. American Journal of Respiratory and Critical Care Medicine. 2011;**183**(10):1419-1426

[53] Rosenzweig I, Glasser M, Crum WR, et al. Changes in neurocognitive architecture in patients with obstructive sleep apnea treated with continuous positive airway pressure. EBioMedicine. 2016;7:221-229

[54] Castronovo V, Scifo P, Castellano A, et al. White matter integrity in obstructive sleep apnea before and after treatment. Sleep. 2014;**37**(9):1465-1475. DOI: 10.5665/sleep.3994

[55] Kim H, Im S, Park J i, et al. Improvement of cognitive function after continuous positive airway pressure treatment for subacute stroke patients with obstructive sleep apnea: A randomized controlled trial. Brain Sciences. 2019;**9**:252

[56] GOLD. Global Strategy for the Diagnosis, Management, and Prevention of Chronic Obstructive Pulmonary Disease: 2019 Report. 2019. Available from: https://goldcopd.org/wp-content/uploads/2018/11/GOLD-2019-v1.7-FINAL-14Nov2018-WMS.pdf

[57] Yohannes AM, Chen W, Moga AM, et al. Cognitive impairment in chronic obstructive pulmonary disease and chronic heart failure: A systematic review and meta-analysis of observational studies. Journal of the American Medical Directors Association;**18**(5):451.e1-451.e11

[58] Oancea C, Tudorache E, Tudorache V. Neurocognitive impairment as systemic effects of COPD. In: McCarthy C, editor. COPD—An Update in Pathogenesis and Clinical Management. 2018;67-86. DOI: 10.5772/intechopen.70580

[59] Crişan AF, Oancea C, Timar B, et al. Cognitive impairment in chronic obstructive pulmonary disease. PLoS One. 2014;**9**(7):e102468

[60] Incalzi RA, Gemma A, Marra C, et al. Chronic obstructive pulmonary disease. An original model of cognitive decline. The American Review of Respiratory Disease. 1993;**148**(2):418-424

[61] Ozge C, Ozge A, Unal O. Cognitive and functional deterioration in patients with severe COPD. Behavioural Neurology. 2006;**17**(2):121-130

[62] Antonelli-Incalzi R, Corsonello A, Pedone C, et al. Drawing impairment predicts mortality in severe COPD. Chest. 2006;**130**(6):1687-1694

[63] Chang SS, Chen S, McAvay GJ, Tinetti ME. Effect of coexisting chronic obstructive pulmonary disease and cognitive impairment on health outcomes in older adults. Journal of the American Geriatrics Society. 2012;**60**:1839-1846

[64] Chen J, Lin IT, Zhang H, et al. Reduced cortical thickness, surface area in patients with chronic obstructive pulmonary disease: A surface-based morphometry and neuropsychological study. Brain Imaging and Behavior. 2016;**10**:464-447

[65] Dodd JW, Getov SV, Jones PW. Cognitive function in COPD. The European Respiratory Journal. 2010;**35**:913-992

[66] Tudorache V, Traila D, Marc M, et al. Impact of moderate to severe obstructive sleep apnea on the cognition in idiopathic pulmonary fibrosis. PLoS One. 2019;**14**(2):e0211455

[67] Pierobon A, Sini Bottelli E, Ranzini L, et al. COPD patients' self-reported adherence, psychosocial factors and mild cognitive impairment in pulmonary rehabilitation. International Journal of Chronic Obstructive Pulmonary Disease. 2017;**12**:2059-2067

[68] Rogliani P, Ora J, Puxeddu E, et al. Adherence to COPD treatment: Myth and reality. Respiratory Medicine. 2017;**129**:117-123

[69] Spruit MA, Singh SJ, Garvey C, et al. An official American Thoracic Society/European Respiratory Society statement: Key concepts and advances in pulmonary rehabilitation. American Journal of Respiratory and Critical Care Medicine. 2013;**188**(8):e13-e64

[70] Chin A, Paw MJM, van Uffelen JGZ, Riphagen I, van Mechelen W. The functional effects of physical exercise training in frail older people. Sports Medicine. 2008;**38**(9):781-793. DOI: 10.2165/00007256-200838090-00006

[71] Palange P, Rohde G, editors. ERS Handbook of Respiratory Medicine. 2019. DOI: 10.1183/9781849840798.erh01. ISBN (electronic): 978-1-84984-079-8

[72] Ley B, Collard HR, King TE Jr. Clinical course and prediction of survival in idiopathic pulmonary fibrosis. American Journal of Respiratory and Critical Care Medicine. 2011;**183**:431-440

[73] Kreuter M, Ehlers-Tenenbaum S, Palmowski K, et al. Impact of comorbidities on mortality in patients with idiopathic pulmonary fibrosis. PLoS One. 2016;**11**(3):e0151425

[74] Raghu G, Amatto VC, Behr J, et al. Comorbidities in idiopathic pulmonary fibrosis patients: A systematic literature review. European Respiratory Journal. 2015;**46**:1113-1130

[75] Oldham JM, Collard HR. Comorbid conditions in idiopathic pulmonary fibrosis: Recognition and management. Frontiers in Medicine (Lausanne). 2017;**4**:123

[76] Javaheri S, Sicilian L. Lung function, breathing pattern, and gas exchange in interstitial lung disease. Thorax. 1992;**47**:93-97

[77] Findley LJ, Ries AL, Tisi GM, et al. Hypoxemia during apnea in normal subjects: Mechanisms and impact of lung volume. Journal of Applied Physiology: Respiratory, Environmental and Exercise Physiology. 1983;**55**:1777-1783

[78] Troy LK, Corte TJ. Sleep disordered breathing in interstitial lung disease: A review. World Journal of Clinical Cases. 2014;**2**:828-834

[79] Pathan SS, Gottesman RF, Mosley TH, et al. Association of lung function with cognitive decline and dementia: The Atherosclerosis Risk in Communities (ARIC) Study. European Journal of Neurology. 2011;**18**:888-898

[80] Lutsey PL, Chen N, Mirabelli MC, et al. Impaired lung function, lung disease and risk of incident dementia. American Journal of Respiratory and Critical Care Medicine. 1 Jun 2019;**199**(11):1385-1396. DOI: 10.1164/rccm.201807-1220OC

[81] Van Dijk EJ, Vermeer SE, de Groot JC, et al. Arterial oxygen saturation, COPD, and cerebral small vessel disease. Journal of Neurology,

Neurosurgery, and Psychiatry. 2004;**75**:733-736

[82] Guo X, Pantoni L, Simoni M, et al. Midlife respiratory function related to white matter lesions and lacunar infarcts in late life. The prospective population study of women in Gothenburg, Sweden. Stroke. 2006;**37**:1658-1662

[83] Yeh H-C, Punjabi NM, Wang N-Y, et al. Vital capacity as a predictor of incident type 2 diabetes: The atherosclerosis risk in communities study. Diabetes Care. 2005;**28**:1472-1479

[84] Schroeder EB, Welch VL, Couper D, et al. Lung functionand incident coronary heart disease: The Atherosclerosis Risk in Communities Study. American Journal of Epidemiology. 2003;**158**:1171-1181

[85] Jiang R, Burke GL, Enright PL, et al. Inflammatory markers and longitudinal lung function decline in the elderly. American Journal of Epidemiology. 2008;**168**:602-610

[86] Schmidt R, Schmidt H, Curb JD, et al. Early inflammation and dementia: A 25-yearfollow-up of the Honolulu-Asia aging study. Annals of Neurology. 2002;**52**:168-174

[87] Sprunger DB, Talbert JL, Brown KK, et al. Cognitive function (CF) is impaired in patients with idiopathic pulmonary fibrosis (IPF). American Journal of Respiratory and Critical Care Medicine. 2009;**179**:A4059. Available from: https://doi.org/10.1164/ajrccm-conference.2009.179.1_MeetingAbstracts.A4059

[88] Sharp C, Adamali H, Millar A, et al. Cognitive function in idiopathic pulmonary fibrosis. Thorax. 2016;**71**:A237

[89] Bors M, Tomic R, Perlman D, et al. Cognitive function in idiopathic pulmonary fibrosis. Chronic Respiratory Disease. 2015;**12**(4):365-372

[90] Nasreddine ZS, Phillips NA, Bédirian V, et al. The Montreal Cognitive Assessment, MoCA: A brief screening tool for mild cognitive impairment. Journal of the American Geriatrics Society. 2005;**53**(4):695-699

[91] Perez-Padilla R, West P, Lertzmann M, et al. Breathing during sleep in patients with interstitial lung disease. The American Review of Respiratory Disease. 1985;**132**:224-229. DOI: 10.1164/arrd.1985.132.2.224

Chapter 4

Presbycusis-Related Tinnitus and Cognitive Impairment: Gender Differences and Common Mechanisms

Weibin Zhang, Zhuowei Yu and Qingwei Ruan

Abstract

Presbycusis-related tinnitus and cognitive impairment are common in the elderly and generate a massive burden on family and society. Except for age, the study explored the gender differences in the prevalence of the three diseases. We found that women have an advantage in maintaining better cognitive and auditory functions. Recent studies suggest the complex links among the three diseases. Peripheral hearing loss can affect sound coding and neural plasticity, which will lead to cognitive impairment and tinnitus. The deficits of the central nervous system, especially central auditory structures, can, in turn, cause the presbycusis. The interaction among three diseases indicated that comprehensive assessment, intervention and treatment in consideration of hearing loss, tinnitus and cognitive impairment are important to decay aging.

Keywords: presbycusis, tinnitus, cognitive impairment, elderly, gender

1. Introduction

Presbycusis-related tinnitus and cognitive impairment are common diseases in the elderly. The three diseases coexist and affect each other.

Presbycusis, also called age-related hearing loss (ARHL), is one of the most frequent hearing disorders among the elderly population. Presbycusis is defined as a bilateral, symmetrical, chronic, and progressive hearing loss, which occurs gradually and initially affects the function of the higher pitched (higher frequency) region [1]. The prevalence of presbycusis is increased rapidly with age increase. Approximately one-third of adults from 61 to 70 years old and more than 80% of populations older than 85 years old in the world complain about the hearing loss [2]. Presbycusis is one of the most common disability conditions, according to the Second China National Census on Disability in 2006. The prevalence of elderly with audition deformity is about 15.4 million, accounting for 34.59% among all types of deformity in people at 60 years and above [3]. Presbycusis is a multifactorial age-related disease that may relate to the interaction among genetic, environmental, and comorbid factors.

Not only the damage of peripheral auditory organs but also the dysfunction of the central auditory nervous system contributes to the sensation of sound.

Therefore, many authors focus on the association between defects in central auditory processing and neurodegenerative diseases [4]. Alzheimer's disease (AD) is the commonest neurodegenerative dementia that occurs in population after 40 years. With the increase of age, the incidence of AD is increased rapidly among the population. Epidemiological surveys show that the prevalence of AD between the ages of 40 and 65 is 1 in 5000 [5]. However, the overall prevalence of dementia increased to 8.5% after 65 years old. By the 85 years old, the prevalence is >20% and creates a devastating burden between family and society [6]. In addition to age, gender, education level, and disease states, such as cardiovascular disease, hyperlipidemia, etc., are all considered as the critical factors of AD [7]. Hearing loss is reported as the independent risk factor for the development of dementia, and 46.4% of dementia was related to hearing loss [8].

Presbycusis can contribute to the emergence of tinnitus. In an epidemiological cohort study, participants were 17% more likely to have tinnitus with every 5-dB increase in pure tone audiometry (PTA) [9]. Tinnitus is charactered as the conscious perception of an abnormal sound in the ears or head either unilaterally or bilaterally, without any external acoustic stimulus [10]. The prevalence of tinnitus increases with increasing age and hearing loss [11, 12]. The etiology of tinnitus remains mostly elusive. Presbycusis-related tinnitus increases cognitive load, including mental balance, attention, concentration, and immediate recall [13]. However, the evidence between tinnitus and cognitive impairment has not been found yet. As lifespans lengthen, the prevalence of elderly populations with presbycusis, dementia, and tinnitus increases rapidly. This review aims to figure out the characters and gender differences of elderly populations with presbycusis-related tinnitus and cognitive impairment and investigate possible mechanisms and treatments.

2. The gender difference in presbycusis

Apart from age, gender seems to be one of the reasons accounting for hearing loss. Numerous epidemiological evidence have suggested that women have better auditory function than men. However, the sexual dimorphism of the function of auditory is tended to converge with aging [14]. Men demonstrate a higher prevalence of presbycusis compared to women. In the 20–69 years old age group, more American men suffer bilateral hearing loss than women [15]. Above 70 years old, men also show independently associated with a higher prevalence of hearing impairment in the United States [16]. For Asian people, similarly, men show higher associated with high frequency hearing loss in the Korean. However, after the age of 60, the level of hearing decline between men and women is similar to age [17]. Pearson et al. found the evidence that the hearing sensitivity decreases with age in both men and women, more rapidly in men than women in young ages or frequencies, in which the decrease begins between age 30 in men and later in women. Though women maintain better auditory function at a young age, they tend to decline fast after menopause. By age 80, the rates of hearing loss are similar between men and women. Sexual dimorphism may be due to the loss of estrogen and progesterone protection [18]. Sexual hormones help women to have benefits in high frequencies. Compared to women at the same age (after menopause), a large cohort study of the healthy population showed that older men had a 10–25 dB worse hearing threshold in the high frequencies [19]. While women have shorter latencies in auditory brainstem response [20], the difference from sex and age cannot be simply explained by the effects of anatomical abnormalities or occupational noise, but it may be related to the decrease of endogenous estrogen that lost the protective effect of estrogen on the auditory system.

3. The gender difference in tinnitus

Elderly Women suffered a lower prevalence of hearing loss and tinnitus loudness than men did, but tinnitus annoyance was stronger in older women than men [21]. However, the underlying mechanism of the difference between men and women is still mysteries. Nondahl et al. reported that an epidemiological cohort study containing 3267 participants from 21 to 84 years old demonstrated that the prevalence of tinnitus was higher for men than for women (11.9 vs. 9.4%, $p = 0.02$), and higher for older (age from 55 to 84 years old) than younger participants (14.4 vs. 9.0%, $p < 0.001$). However, adjusted for factors related to tinnitus, it showed no association between sex and tinnitus [9]. An epidemiological study of 6333 population in China showed no significant difference in prevalence between men and women age >60 years [22]. For the loudness of tinnitus, some found a low correlation of gender [23], while others reported significantly higher loudness in men compared to women. However, older women tend to report a higher level of an emotional reaction than men with tinnitus [20] and frequently more severe, accompanied by vertigo [24].

4. The gender difference in cognitive impairment

The majority of epidemiological research indicated that women with aging are sensitive to dementia even after controlling for increased life span and education level, which show a rapid decline in a cognitive deterioration compared with age-matched men [25]. The animal experiment indicated that follicular depletion might initiate age-related impairments for cognitive flexibility [26]. The postmenopausal women have a two-fold higher lifetime risk of developing AD than men and demonstrate a faster cognition decline [27, 28]. However, some clinical evidence show that older women performed better on the global function test while men at the same age on the executive function test, respectively [29], and found more significant risk for men [30]. Other studies suggested that gender does not play a role in the prevalence of AD [31, 32].

5. The association between presbycusis and tinnitus

Several researches suggest that hearing loss contributes to the higher prevalence of tinnitus [33]. At present, the following two reasons are mostly considered. One reason is the sensory deprivation of the auditory system. The decrease in auditory stimulation leads to the unbalance between excitation and inhibition in the auditory nervous system [34]. The auditory nervous system has both suppression and excitation response region. Once a sound is inputted, excitation action will be activated and lateral inhibition appears consequently. Hearing loss reduces the activity of cochlear and downregulates inhibitory neurons processes, thereby activating the central auditory structures, increasing the spontaneous firing rate of neurons, resulting in the awareness of tinnitus. Sound stimulation at different frequencies can inhibit the formation of tinnitus. Studies have shown that high frequency sounds have a stronger suppression of tinnitus, and the decline of high frequency is a common and typical symptom in the ARHL [35]. The activation of neural plasticity in the central auditory system plays a vital role in maintaining the sensory of tinnitus [36]. Because when the auditory nerve was removed, the tinnitus persists [37]. Neural plasticity can change the processing of sounds, reroute auditory signals in the central nervous system, increase neural synchrony, and promote coherent firings of activity in many neurons [38]. Another reason is that hearing loss and tinnitus share the same common risks, including age, cardiovascular disorders, and noise exposure [39].

6. The association between presbycusis and cognitive decline

Clinically, patients with presbycusis usually perform worse than others in function of speech and communication, resulting in negative psychosocial endings such as social isolation and social frailty [40]; depression, poor cognitive performance and even induce cognitive decline [33, 41]; and low physical performance and physical frailty [42, 43]. A meta-analysis of 36 epidemiological studies and 20,264 participants showed that the decline of cognitive domains are significantly associated with ARHL [44]. Hearing loss is considered as the independent risk factor for the development of dementia, and 46.4% of patients with dementia were accompanying hearing loss [8]. There may be a bidirectional connection between presbycusis and dementia. On the one hand, it is more likely for the elderly with hearing impairment to suffer dementia than the healthy elderly [45], and on the other hand, the hearing threshold of the elderly with dementia is significantly lower than the healthy elderly [45–47]. A large cross-sectional study in the UK shows the association between hearing aid use with better cognitive function [48]. The hearing intervention significantly improves the auditory and cognitive function in the elderly [49].

Presbycusis and dementia may share some common pathophysiological mechanisms [50, 51] once degradation on one pathway may accelerate the degradation on each other disease. The hypothetical mechanistic pathways are still uncertain. However, some authors may agree that hearing loss can impair speech perception and distort peripheral encoding of sound by the cochlea. Besides, peripheral hearing loss has a negative influence on the measurements or process of central auditory; finally, it increases cognitive load, depletes cognitive reserve, alters brain structure and function, and affects global cognition [52, 53]. Hearing loss will cause social isolation and loneliness associated with chronic stress and depression. The psychosocial outcomes contribute to hippocampal atrophy and cognitive decline through the hypothalamic-pituitary-adrenal (HPA) axis [8, 54]. The dysfunction of HPA axis results in the atrophy of pyramidal cell dendrites, thereby reducing the ability of hippocampal structural plasticity and synapse generation.

7. The association between cognitive decline and tinnitus

Little research focuses on the association between presbycusis co-occurring with tinnitus and dementia. However, central nervous degenerative diseases such as dementia will affect central auditory systems (i.e., temporal and adjacent frontal lobes) and cause central auditory disorders, which is an essential physiological pathway of the diseases. Not only the central auditory structure but also the non-auditory brain areas (i.e., frontal cortex or the limbic system) play a vital role in sound perception, understanding, and emotional awareness [55]. Inflammation and ischemia will cause disturbances to the central nervous system [56]. When the neural substrates of tinnitus (i.e., medial temporal lobe, primary auditory, and frontal cortices) are involved, tinnitus and hearing allergies occur [57]. Meanwhile, inflammation and ischemia can develop neurodegeneration disease of AD in frontoparietotemporal [58]. AD shares the same pathological basis with tinnitus, although targets in different areas. On the other hand, chronic tinnitus is significantly associated with anxiety and depression. The limbic system was proved to contribute to the emotional burden. Presbycusis co-occurring with tinnitus may accompany vestibular/balance difficulties, similar to anxiety and depression; it will reduce social activity and finally leads to late-life cognitive decline [53].

8. The treatments in the coexistence of presbycusis-related tinnitus and cognitive impairment

Presbycusis-related tinnitus and cognitive impairment are complex diseases without any effective treatment by far. However, compared to age-matched men, women before menopause seem to have a better auditory and cognitive function, while the different fades away with age. Sex hormones may play an important role. The association among the diseases indicates the feasibility of intervening in the hearing loss to ameliorate the tinnitus and cognitive impairment. A comprehensive assessment is a prerequisite for treatment. Hearing aid and cochlear implantation are the most important treatment of hearing loss.

Emerging studies suggest that the use of hearing aid or cochlear implants can not only focus on auditory rehabilitation but also improve the symptom of cognitive function and tinnitus [59–62]. However, the prevalence of hearing aid use is low [63]. Only 14.2% of Americans 50 years old with hearing loss wear hearing aids, not to mention the populations in developing countries [64]. Many patients with hearing loss tend to ignore the hearing loss as normal aging until the accelerated deterioration of the auditory function. Furthermore, the expensive cost of hearing aid and cochlear implantation hold back the eager of intervention.

In turn, advanced technology and equipment (i.e., virtually reality) can be designed to improve cognitive function and central auditory disorder through reasonable and repeated cognitive and behavioral treatment for functions such as sensation, cognition, emotion, and motor control [65, 66].

9. Conclusion

Presbycusis-related tinnitus and dementia are a common disturbance to the elderly but always be unnoticed at an early stage. Age is the most important factor for the diseases. Apart from age, most epidemiological evidence suggest that women have a better auditory and cognitive function and less prevalence of tinnitus than men; however, the advantages disappear with age. The three diseases interact and promote each other with decreased peripheral hearing perception and central nervous system dysfunction. The elderly should pay attention to auditory function carefully. Maintaining normal peripheral and central auditory function can reduce cognitive decline and tinnitus. Conversely, the elderly with cognitive decline or tinnitus should actively participate in cognitive and behavioral treatment to enhance central auditory function.

Acknowledgements

This work was supported by the Medical Science and Technology Support Project of Shanghai Science and Technology Commission (18411962200), Shanghai Center for Clinical Medicine and Key Discipline Construction (2017ZZ02010).

Author details

Weibin Zhang, Zhuowei Yu and Qingwei Ruan*
Shanghai Key Laboratory of Clinical Geriatrics, Shanghai Institute of Geriatrics and Gerontology, Huadong Hospital and Research Center of Aging and Medicine, Shanghai Medical College, Fudan University, Shanghai, P.R. China

*Address all correspondence to: 13661717346@163.com

References

[1] Fetoni AR, Picciotti PM, Paludetti G, et al. Pathogenesis of presbycusis in animal models: A review. Experimental Gerontology. 2011;**46**(6):413-425. DOI: 10.1016/j.exger.2010.12.003

[2] Fortunato S, Forli F, Guglielmi V, et al. A review of new insights on the association between hearing loss and cognitive decline in ageing. Acta Otorhinolaryngologica Italica. 2016;**36**(3):155-166. DOI: 10.14639/0392-100x-993

[3] Yu L, Sun X, Wei Z, et al. A study on the status quo of aged population with hearing loss in China. Chinese Scientific Journal of Hearing and Speech Rehabilitation. 2008;**3**:63-65

[4] Ruan Q, Cheng M, Zhang R, Yu Z. Current status of auditory aging and anti-aging research. Geriatrics and Gerontology International. 2013;**14**:40-53

[5] Renvoize E, Hanson M, Dale M. Prevalence and causes of young onset dementia in an English health district. International Journal of Geriatric Psychiatry. 2011;**26**(1):106-107

[6] Koller D, Bynum JPW. Dementia in the USA: State variation in prevalence. Journal of Public Health. 2014;**37**(4)

[7] Sjogren M, Mielke M, Gustafson D, et al. Cholesterol and Alzheimer's disease—Is there a relation? Mechanisms of Ageing and Development. 2006;**127**(2):138-147. DOI: 10.1016/j.mad.2005.09.020

[8] Lin FR, Metter EJ, O'Brien RJ, et al. Hearing loss and incident dementia. Archives of Neurology. 2011;**68**(2):214-220. DOI: 10.1001/archneurol.2010.362

[9] Nondahl DM, Cruickshanks KJ, Huang GH, et al. Tinnitus and its risk factors in the beaver dam offspring study. International Journal of Audiology. 2011;**50**(5):313-320. DOI: 10.3109/14992027.2010.551220

[10] Martini A, Castiglione A, Bovo R, et al. Aging, cognitive load, dementia and hearing loss. Audiology and Neuro-Otology. 2014;**19**(Suppl 1):2-5. DOI: 10.1159/000371593

[11] Baguley DM. Mechanisms of tinnitus. British Medical Bulletin. 2002;**63**:195-212

[12] Shargorodsky J, Curhan GC, Farwell WR. Prevalence and characteristics of tinnitus among US adults. The American Journal of Medicine. 2010;**123**(8):711-718. DOI: 10.1016/j.amjmed.2010.02.015

[13] Gudwani S, Munjal SK, Panda NK, et al. Association of chronic subjective tinnitus with neuro-cognitive performance. The International Tinnitus Journal. 2017;**21**(2):90-97. DOI: 10.5935/0946-5448.20170018

[14] Homans NC, Metselaar RM, Dingemanse JG, et al. Prevalence of age-related hearing loss, including sex differences, in older adults in a large cohort study. The Laryngoscope. 2017;**127**(3):725-730. DOI: 10.1002/lary.26150

[15] Agrawal Y, Platz EA, Niparko JK. Prevalence of hearing loss and differences by demographic characteristics among US adults: Data from the National Health and Nutrition Examination Survey, 1999-2004. Archives of Internal Medicine. 2008;**168**(14):1522-1530. DOI: 10.1001/archinte.168.14.1522

[16] Lin FR, Thorpe R, Gordon-Salant S, et al. Hearing loss prevalence and risk factors among older adults in the United States. Journal of Gerontology. 2011;**66**(5):582

[17] Hong JW, Jeon JH, Ku CR, et al. The prevalence and factors associated with hearing impairment in the Korean adults. Medicine (Baltimore). 2015;**94**(10):e611. DOI: 10.1097/MD.0000000000000611

[18] Pearson JD, Morrell CH, Gordon-Salant S, et al. Gender differences in a longitudinal study of age-associated hearing loss. The Journal of the Acoustical Society of America. 1995;**97**(2):1196-1205

[19] Jonsson R, Rosenhall U, Gause-Nilsson I, et al. Auditory function in 70- and 75-year-olds of four age cohorts. A cross-sectional and time-lag study of presbyacusis. Scandinavian Audiology. 1998;**27**(2):81-93

[20] Jerger J, Hall J. Effects of age and sex on auditory brainstem response. Archives of Otolaryngology—Head and Neck Surgery. 1980;**106**(7):387-391

[21] Seydel C, Haupt H, Olze H, et al. Gender and chronic tinnitus: Differences in tinnitus-related distress depend on age and duration of tinnitus. Ear and Hearing. 2013;**34**(5):661-672. DOI: 10.1097/AUD.0b013e31828149f2

[22] Xu X, Bu X, Zhou L, et al. An epidemiologic study of tinnitus in a population in Jiangsu Province, China. Journal of the American Academy of Audiology. 2011;**22**(9):578-585. DOI: 10.3766/jaaa.22.9.3

[23] Seimetz BM, Teixeira AR, Rosito LPS, et al. Pitch and loudness tinnitus in individuals with Presbycusis. International Archives of Otorhinolaryngology. 2016;**20**(4):321-326. DOI: 10.1055/s-0035-1570311

[24] Ferreira LMDBM, Mendes EP. Characterization of tinnitus in the elderly and its possible related disorders. Brazilian Journal of Otorhinolaryngology. 2009;**75**(2):249-255

[25] Li R, Singh M. Sex differences in cognitive impairment and Alzheimer's disease. Frontiers in Neuroendocrinology. 2014;**35**(3):385-403. DOI: 10.1016/j.yfrne.2014.01.002

[26] Koebele SV, Mennenga SE, Hiroi R, et al. Cognitive changes across the menopause transition: A longitudinal evaluation of the impact of age and ovarian status on spatial memory. Hormones and Behavior. 2017;**87**:96-114. DOI: 10.1016/j.yhbeh.2016.10.010

[27] Laws KR, Irvine K, Gale TM. Sex differences in cognitive impairment in Alzheimer's disease. World Journal of Psychiatry. 2016;**6**(1):54-65

[28] Zagni E, Simoni L, Colombo D. Sex and gender differences in central nervous system-related disorders. Neuroscience Journal. 2016;**2016**(2):1-13

[29] Reas ET, Laughlin GA, Bergstrom J, et al. Effects of sex and education on cognitive change over a 27-year period in older adults: The rancho Bernardo study. The American Journal of Geriatric Psychiatry: Official Journal of the American Association for Geriatric Psychiatry. 2017;**25**(8):889-899. DOI: 10.1016/j.jagp.2017.03.008

[30] Petersen RC, Roberts RO, Knopman DS, et al. Prevalence of mild cognitive impairment is higher in men: The Mayo Clinic study of aging. Neurology. 2010;**75**(10):889-897

[31] Ruitenberg A, Ott A, Swieten JCV, et al. Incidence of dementia: Does gender make a difference? Neurobiology of Aging. 2001;**22**(4):575-580

[32] Solfrizzi V, Panza F, Colacicco AM, et al. Vascular risk factors, incidence of MCI, and rates of progression to dementia. Neurology. 2004;**63**(10):1882-1891

[33] Haider HF, Flook M, Aparicio M, et al. Biomarkers of Presbycusis and

tinnitus in a Portuguese older population. Frontiers in Aging Neuroscience. 2017;**9**:346. DOI: 10.3389/fnagi.2017.00346

[34] Eggermont JJ, Roberts LE. The neuroscience of tinnitus. Trends in Neurosciences. 2004;**27**(11):0-682

[35] Møller AR. The role of auditory deprivation. In: Textbook of Tinnitus. New York: Springer; 2011. pp. 95-99

[36] Noreña AJ, Eggermont JJ. Changes in spontaneous neural activity immediately after an acoustic trauma: Implications for neural correlates of tinnitus. Hearing Research;**183**(1-2):0-153

[37] House JW, Brackmann DE. Tinnitus: Surgical treatment. In: Ciba Foundation Symposium. John Wiley & Sons, Ltd; 2008

[38] Seki S, Eggermont JJ. Changes in spontaneous firing rate and neural synchrony in cat primary auditory cortex after localized tone-induced hearing loss. Hearing Research;**180**(1-2):0-38

[39] Møller AR. Epidemiology of tinnitus in adults. In: Textbook of Tinnitus. New York: Springer; 2011. pp. 29-39

[40] Bunt S, Steverink N, Olthof J, et al. Social frailty in older adults: A scoping review. European Journal of Ageing. 2017;**14**(3):1-12

[41] Gates GA, Cobb JL, Linn RT, et al. Central auditory dysfunction, cognitive dysfunction, and dementia in older people. Archives of Otolaryngology—Head and Neck Surgery. 1996;**122**(2):161-167

[42] Karpa MJ, Gopinath B, Beath K, et al. Associations between hearing impairment and mortality risk in older persons: The Blue Mountains hearing study. Annals of Epidemiology. 2010;**20**(6):452-459

[43] Liljas AEM, Carvalho LA, Papachristou E, et al. Self-reported hearing impairment and incident frailty in English community-dwelling older adults: A 4-year follow-up study. Journal of the American Geriatrics Society. 2017;**65**(5):958-965

[44] Loughrey DG, Kelly ME, Kelley GA, et al. Association of age-related hearing loss with cognitive function, cognitive impairment, and dementia: A systematic review and meta-analysis. JAMA Otolaryngology. Head and Neck Surgery. 2017;**144**(2):115-126

[45] Panza F, Solfrizzi V, Logroscino G. Age-related hearing impairment-a risk factor and frailty marker for dementia and AD. Nature Reviews Neurology. 2015;**11**(3):166-175. DOI: 10.1038/nrneurol.2015.12

[46] Lin FR. Hearing loss and cognition among older adults in the United States. The Journals of Gerontology Series A, Biological Sciences and Medical Sciences. 2011;**66**(10):1131-1136. DOI: 10.1093/gerona/glr115

[47] Lin FR, Ferrucci L, Metter EJ, et al. Hearing loss and cognition in the Baltimore longitudinal study of aging. Neuropsychology. 2011;**25**(6):763-770. DOI: 10.1037/a0024238

[48] Piers D, Richard E, CK J, et al. Hearing loss and cognition: The role of hearing aids, social isolation and depression. PLoS One;**10**(3):e0119616

[49] Deal JA, Albert MS, Arnold M, et al. A randomized feasibility pilot trial of hearing treatment for reducing cognitive decline: Results from the aging and cognitive health evaluation in elders pilot study. Alzheimer's and Dementia (New York). 2017;**3**(3):410-415. DOI: 10.1016/j.trci.2017.06.003

[50] Ronnberg J, Danielsson H, Rudner M, et al. Hearing loss is negatively related to episodic and

semantic long-term memory but not to short-term memory. Journal of Speech, Language, and Hearing Research: JSLHR. 2011;**54**(2):705-726. DOI: 10.1044/1092-4388(2010/09-0088)

[51] Ruan Q, Yu Z, Zhang W, et al. Cholinergic hypofunction in presbycusis-related tinnitus with cognitive function impairment: Emerging hypotheses. Frontiers in Aging Neuroscience. 2018;**10**:98

[52] Lin FR, Albert M. Hearing loss and dementia—Who is listening? Aging and Mental Health. 2014;**18**(6):671-673

[53] Rutherford BR, Brewster K, Golub JS, et al. Sensation and psychiatry: Linking age-related hearing loss to late-life depression and cognitive decline. The American Journal of Psychiatry. 2018;**175**(3):215-224

[54] Ruan Q, D'Onofrio G, Wu T, et al. Sexual dimorphism of frailty and cognitive impairment: Potential underlying mechanisms (review). Molecular Medicine Reports. 2017;**16**(3):3023-3033

[55] Mahoney C, Rossor MN, Rohrer JD, et al. POD07 tinnitus and hyperacusis in semantic dementia. Journal of Neurology, Neurosurgery and Psychiatry. 2010;**81**:e43-e44

[56] Shulman A, Goldstein B, Strashun AM. Central nervous system neurodegeneration and tinnitus: A clinical experience. Part II: Translational neurovascular theory of neurodegenerative CNS disease and tinnitus. The International Tinnitus Journal. 2008;**14**(1):43

[57] Mahoney CJ, Rohrer JD, Goll JC, et al. Structural neuroanatomy of tinnitus and hyperacusis in semantic dementia. Journal of Neurology, Neurosurgery, and Psychiatry. 2011;**82**(11):1274-1278

[58] Bailey TL, Rivara CB, Rocher AB, et al. The nature and effects of cortical microvascular pathology in aging and Alzheimer's disease. Neurological Research. 2004;**26**(5):573-578

[59] Beck LD. Hearing aid amplification and tinnitus: 2011 overview. Hearing Journal;**64**(6):12-14

[60] Castiglione A, Benatti A, Velardita C, et al. Aging, cognitive decline and hearing loss: Effects of auditory rehabilitation and training with hearing aids and cochlear implants on cognitive function and depression among older adults. Audiology and Neuro-Otology. 2016;**21**(1):21-28

[61] Strauss DJ, Corona-Strauss FI, Seidler H, et al. Notched environmental sounds: A new hearing aid supported tinnitus treatment evaluated in 20 patients. Clinical Otolaryngology. 2017;**42**(1):172-175

[62] Heyning PVD, Vermeire K, Diebl M, et al. Incapacitating unilateral tinnitus in single-sided deafness treated by cochlear implantation. The Annals of Otology, Rhinology, and Laryngology. 2008;**117**(9):645-652

[63] Popelka MM, Cruickshanks KJ, Wiley TL, et al. Low prevalence of hearing aid use among older adults with hearing loss: The epidemiology of hearing loss study. Journal of the American Geriatrics Society;**46**(9):1075-1078

[64] Chien W, Lin FR. Prevalence of hearing aid use among older adults in the United States. Archives of Internal Medicine. 2012;**172**(3):292-293

[65] Yu Z, Zhang W, Jian R, et al. Chapter 1 virtual reality in the assessment and rehabilitation of the elderly population with physical and cognitive impairment. In: Active & Healthy Aging: Novel Robotic Solutions

and Internet of Things. Avid Science; 2017. pp. 1-44

[66] Mahncke HW, Bronstone A, Merzenich MM. Brain plasticity and functional losses in the aged: Scientific bases for a novel intervention. Progress in Brain Research. 2006;**157**:81-109

Chapter 5

Audiovestibular Dysfunction and Hearing Loss in Patients with Psoriasis and Psoriatic Arthritis

Sevgi Akarsu

Abstract

Psoriasis is now considered a T cell-mediated chronic systemic inflammatory disease rather than only a simple skin disease. The relationship and coexistence of this common disease with many other comorbidities have gained increasing attention in recent years. Although psoriatic skin lesions are seen frequently in the auricle and external auditory canal, there are not many studies evaluating the possible effect of psoriatic disease (psoriasis with or without joint involvement) on the auditory system. Hearing impairment detected in psoriasis patients is mostly seen as subclinical hearing loss at high frequencies, but it can also have a significant impact on patients' health and quality of life due to the possible risk of developing sudden sensorineural hearing loss. In this chapter, the frequency, pattern, and patient-related risk factors of hearing impairment and audiovestibular dysfunction in patients with psoriasis and psoriatic arthritis were extensively reviewed and discussed. In conclusion, it was emphasized that subclinical sensorineural hearing loss is a neglected but an important comorbidity in patients with psoriasis and psoriatic arthritis. The relationship between psoriatic disease and audiovestibular dysfunction supports the need for further studies aimed at better identification of the underlying pathogenic mechanisms, and accordingly to update diagnostic and even treatment approaches.

Keywords: psoriasis, psoriatic arthritis, hearing impairment, sensorineural hearing loss, deafness, audiovestibular dysfunction

1. Introduction

Psoriasis is a common erythemato-squamous disease which has a prevalence of 2–4% in the general population [1, 2]. Even though the precise etiology remains unknown, it is now considered an autoimmune, chronic, immune-mediated inflammatory disease (IMID) characterized by T cell mediated hyperproliferation of keratinocytes [3, 4]. There are multiple clinical types of psoriasis that can overlap in a spectrum from mild sebopsoriasis localized to the scalp to generalized pustular psoriasis. In the most common type of psoriasis vulgaris, the diameters of erythemato-squamous papular lesions can range from pinhead-size to plaques covering the larger skin surface. Besides typical skin involvement in psoriasis, significant deterioration of the nails and painful inflammatory joint involvement (psoriatic arthritis, PsA) can also be seen [1, 2]. PsA is a disease in the group of seronegative

IntechOpen

spondyloarthropathies, such as ankylosing spondylitis and reactive arthritis. While its prevalence in the general population has been estimated between 0.02% and 0.42%, its frequency in people with psoriasis ranges from 6–42%. This inflammatory arthritis has different symptoms such as pain, swelling or stiffness and sausage digits (dactylitis) in one or more joints, Achilles tendinitis or plantar fasciitis. Psoriasis and PsA have been considered by some clinicians as different diseases due to various diagnostic criteria and different clinical courses, but the relationship between both diseases cannot be ignored [5–7]. It is well known that psoriatic disease with or without arthritis can occur at any age and negatively affects the quality of life by disrupting lifelong physical and psychosocial health [8, 9].

External ear involvement is also common in psoriasis [10]. Approximately two-thirds of patients have typical psoriatic lesions characterized by itchy, well-demarcated, erythemato-squamous plaques on the earlobe and conchal bowl. Although non-specific erythematous, scaly and dry lesions are sometimes seen in the ear, the precise diagnosis of ear psoriasis can be made easily by detecting typical psoriatic lesions in other areas of the body [2, 11]. Despite the high prevalence of clinical lesions affecting the auricle and the external auditory canal in psoriasis, there are not many studies evaluating the possible effect of psoriatic disease on the auditory system [12–25]. The auricle and outer one-third of the external auditory canal contain elastic cartilage covered with skin and its appendages, including mainly hair cells, and sebaceous and apocrine glands. It has been reported that chronic cutaneous inflammation and keratinocyte hyperproliferation induce progressive skin thickening with the tendency of substenosis and serum accumulation in the external auditory canal and stenosis of the tympanic membrane, causing disruption in sound transmission to the middle ear [22]. It is also well known that otitis externa is frequently seen in infection-prone conditions such as psoriasis [10]. Moreover, the rare ototoxic effect of topical salicylic acid, which is among the antipsoriatic topical treatments, was reported in a few cases. Maune et al. observed recurrent, symmetrical, pancochlear, reversible inner ear failure in a psoriasis patient using topical salicylate [26]. However, for the first time in 2004, sudden-onset autoimmune sensorineural hearing loss (SNHL) was reported in two cases with PsA [27, 28]. Yen et al. evaluated the risk of sudden SNHL in patients with psoriasis in a retrospective cohort study involving 28.817 patients and gender-, age-, and comorbidities-matched controls. The incidence of sudden SNHL was found about 1.51 times higher in the psoriasis cohort after 6 years of follow-up than in the control cohort [12].

In previous studies, it has been mentioned that the inner ear is sensitive to local or systemic autoimmune attacks and SNHL can occur as a complication of non-organ-specific autoimmune diseases [29–32]. The hypothesis that SNHL may develop as a result of an autoimmune process against the inner ear was first introduced by Lehnhardt in 1958 [33]. 20 years later (1979), McCabe was the first to describe SNHL that may occur in the autoimmune diseases. The idea was suggested by the author that an autoimmune pathogenesis may be present in the etiology upon improvement of hearing after corticosteroid therapy in a patient with progressive bilateral idiopathic SNHL [34]. Since then, several cases of SNHL and acute/subclinical audiovestibular dysfunction accompanied by various autoimmune and autoinflammatory diseases including vitiligo, inflammatory bowel disease (e.g., Crohn's disease, ulcerative colitis), Behçet's disease, Wegener's granulomatosis, rheumatoid arthritis, systemic lupus erythematosus, Sjogren's syndrome, relapsing polychondritis, giant cell arteritis, ankylosing spondylitis, Vogt-Koyanagi-Harada syndrome, Cogan's syndrome and Susac's syndrome, have been reported in the literature [29, 35, 36]. Current literature information shows that SNHL is the most common auditory symptom of systemic autoimmune diseases, but due to the different presentations (sudden or progressive) and severity (mild or severe) of SNHL, early correlation between symptom and systemic autoimmune disease may be difficult [29]. Additionally, audiovestibular symptoms found in autoimmune conditions are also common in other disorders, such as diabetes and hypertension. For these reasons, the correct differential diagnosis of the cause of audiovestibular involvement is very important [30, 31].

Although autoimmunity has been accused of sudden hearing loss for many years, interest in studies related to the inner ear involvement secondary to systemic autoimmune diseases has been gradually increasing in recent years [30, 35]. In the literature about psoriatic disease-related hearing loss, firstly, Srikumar et al. reported a 62-year-old male patient with PsA, who had been under methotrexate therapy, developed sudden onset of SNHL and recovered with oral corticosteroids. So that, it was suggested by the author that PsA should have added to autoimmune diseases that can cause SNHL [27]. Subsequently, Giani et al. reported the development of bilateral asymmetric sensorineural deafness, which improved with oral prednisolone without interruption of previous etanercept therapy, in a 13-year-old girl with juvenile PsA [28]. However, after these case reports, a limited number of studies evaluating hearing and/or the audiovestibular system were conducted to determine whether the chronic inflammatory process and/or autoimmunity affect the inner ear in psoriasis patients with or without joint involvement [12–25].

In this chapter, case reports, clinical trials, cohort studies, systematic reviews and meta-analyses associated with hearing impairment and audiovestibular dysfunction in patients with psoriasis and PsA published up until now were comprehensively reviewed and discussed. The Medline literature database was searched through PubMed using the keywords, individually and in combination: 'psoriasis', 'psoriatic arthritis', 'hearing loss', 'sensorineural hearing loss', 'deafness', 'hearing impairment' and 'audiovestibular dysfunction'. Only articles available in original or translated English were evaluated.

2. Audiological/audiovestibular evaluations in patients with psoriasis/psoriatic arthritis

When all clinical studies are reviewed, it has been observed that psoriasis/PsA patients and the control group consisting of volunteer healthy subjects were compared with each other in terms of audiological changes [12–25]. In just a few studies, these groups were also evaluated in terms of the accompanying vestibular system involvement [15, 20, 21, 25]. Comprehensive ear, nose and throat examinations were performed by otorhinolaryngologists in all cases before audiological evaluations. Subsequently, pure tone audiometric and otoacoustic emission (distortion product or transient evoked) tests, as well vestibular tests in some studies were applied by audiometrists (**Table 1**). Generally, cases with the current and/or past history of chronic otitis externa, recurrent otitis media, inner ear infections, otosclerosis, suppurative labyrinthitis, Meniere disease and other vestibular syndromes, congenital ear disease, ear membrane perforation, ear surgery, head and neck trauma, exposure to high-decibel levels, cardiovascular disease (ischemic heart disease including angina, myocardial infarction, heart failure), cerebrovascular events (transient ischemic attacks/strokes confirmed by MRI/CT brain scan), peripheral arterial disease confirmed by Doppler ultrasound and/or arteriography, renal insufficiency, vertigo, any ototoxic drug use (e.g., quinolones, macrolides, aminoglycosides, antidepressants, beta blockers, hormone antagonists, antiglaucoma preparations, antimalarials), flat tympanogram and hearing aid use were not included in these studies. It was observed that current and/or past use of

References	Study cases	Audiological/audiovestibular diagnostic tests
[13]	42 PSO patients, 60 healthy controls	Pure tone audiometry (0.25, 0.5, 1, 2, 4, 6 kHz) Tympanometry, Acoustic reflex Distortion product otoacoustic emission testing
[14]	51 PSO patients, 51 healthy controls	Pure tone audiometry
[15]	60 PsA patients, 60 matched controls	Pure tone audiometry (0.5, 1, 2, 3, 4, 6, 8 kHz) Speech discrimination test, tympanometry, stapedius reflex threshold MRI of the posterior fossa and brainstem Videonystagmography testing device Spontaneous nystagmus, gaze-evoked nystagmus, oculocephalic response, head-shaking nystagmus Oculographic tests (saccades; slow, smooth pursuit evaluation; and optokinetic stimulus) Positional nystagmus in supine, lying on the right, lying on the left, and cervical hyperextension positions (head hanging) Cephalic rotational test in the supine position; Dix-Hallpike test Quantitative postural function test Bithermal water caloric test
[16]	31 PsA patients, 31 healthy controls	Pure tone audiometry (0.25, 0.5, 1, 2, 4, 6 kHz) Speech discrimination score, tympanometry Transient evoked otoacoustic emissions
[17]	41 PSO patients, 41 healthy controls	Pure tone audiometry (air-conduction at 0.25, 0.5, 1, 2, 4, 8 kHz; bone-conduction at 0.5, 1, 2, 4 kHz) Transient evoked otoacoustic emissions
[18]	24 PsA patients, 38 healthy controls	Distortion product otoacoustic emissions (1–4 kHz) Tympanometric examination Stapes reflex values, speech reception threshold Speech discrimination values Pure tone values (0.25 kHz – 8 kHz) High-frequency values (10, 12.5, 16 kHz)
[19]	50 PSO patients, 45 healthy controls	Pure tone audiogram (0.5 kHz –16 kHz) Speech audiometry
[20]	60 PsA patients, 60 matched controls	Clinical test of sensory integration and balance Computerized dynamic posturography
[21]	61 PSO patients, 61 healthy controls	Pure tone audiometry (0.25–1 kHz, 2–6 kHz), autoacoustic emission, stapes reflex, detection threshold of speech - discrimination Electronystagmography tests; spontaneous nystagmus, gaze-evoked nystagmus, oculographic tests (saccades; slow, smooth pursuit evaluation; optokinetic stimulus) Positional nystagmus in supine, lying on the right, lying on the left, cervical hyperextension positions (head hanging) Cephalic rotational test in the supine position Dix-Hallpike test, Bi-thermal water caloric test
[22]	77 PSO patients, 77 healthy controls	Tympanometry Audiometric tests
[23]	29 PSO patients, 30 healthy controls	Tympanography Pure tone audiometry (0.25, 0.5, 1, 2, 4, 8, 10, 12, 14, 16 kHz) Speech audiometry, impedance audiometry Transient evoked otoacoustic emissions Distortion product otoacoustic emissions
[24]	50 PSO patients, 50 healthy controls	Pure tone audiometry (0.25, 0.5, 1, 2, 4, 8 kHz)

References	Study cases	Audiological/audiovestibular diagnostic tests
[25]	32 PSO patients (−) arthritis, 35 healthy controls	Pure tone audiometry (0.25, 0.5, 1, 2, 4, 6, 8 kHz) Distortion product otoacoustic emission (2,3,4,5 kHz) Spontaneous and gaze-evoked nystagmus Head shake test, tandem stance test, Unterberger test, Romberg test, Dix-Hallpike test, supine roll test, head hanging test Oculomotor and caloric tests

PSO (Psoriasis); PsA (Psoriatic Arthritis).

Table 1.
Audiological/audiovestibular diagnostic tests in patients with psoriasis/psoriatic arthritis.

non-steroidal anti-inflammatory drugs, prednisone, methotrexate and/or tumor necrosis factor-α (TNF-α) antagonists were present in all patients with PsA and in some psoriasis patients. To evaluate the clinical severity of psoriatic disease, mostly Psoriasis Area and Severity Index (PASI) was used. In addition to PASI, body surface area, investigator's global assessment and dermatology life quality index were applied in a few studies [13–25]. The results of these studies are summarized below in chronological order.

Firstly, Karabulut et al. (2010) did not find a statistically significant difference between each groups for either pure tone audiometric hearing thresholds or distortion product autoacustic emissions in a case-control study involving 42 patients with psoriasis. In addition, neither SNHL nor any damage of outer hair cells of cochlea was detected. The authors suggested that the increase in the frequency of hearing loss and vestibular disorders in chronic inflammatory and autoimmune diseases may be due to the more prominent role of CD4 T cells rather than the predominant CD8 T cells in psoriasis [13].

In 2012, Guvenc et al.'s study (involving 51 psoriasis patients, 51 controls) demonstrated that the hearing threshold values at all frequencies for air conduction and bone conduction in psoriasis patients were significantly higher than in the control group with the pure tone audiometry measurements. Statistical significance was achieved in all frequencies (more pronounced at higher frequencies) except to right ear air conduction 1000 Hz, bone conduction 500 and 1000 Hz, as well left ear air conduction 500 Hz and bone conduction 500 Hz measurements. No significant relationship was found in the correlation analysis between age and psoriasis duration and hearing loss. When the PASI score adjusted for age and disease duration and threshold values matching the frequencies were compared with the correlation analysis, a significant correlation was found between the PASI score and hearing loss at medium and high frequencies. The fact that the hearing loss detected was independent of age and disease duration suggested to the authors that hearing loss in psoriasis is not an age-related degeneration and is not due to the long-term low-level effect of inflammatory mediators. Due to the statistically significant and moderately correlation between hearing loss at medium and high frequencies (bone conduction 2000, 4000 Hz; air conduction 1000, 2000, 4000, 8000 Hz) and high PASI scores, the authors considered that hearing loss is occurred as a consequence of increasing proinflammatory cytokines such as TNF-α (which is responsible for the severity of the psoriatic disease) in exacerbation periods of psoriasis and subsequently causing cochlear degeneration [14].

A case-control study of 60 PsA patients by Amor-Dorado et al. (2014) demonstrated that the frequencies of tinnitus, vertigo and disequilibrium as well as the subjective hearing loss (31.7% of PsA vs. 6.7% of controls) were significantly higher in the PsA group. Patients with PsA exhibited significantly higher values of pure tone audiogram and speech reception threshold than controls. Abnormal hearing loss in the audiogram (60% vs. 8.3%), bilateral and symmetrical SNHL predominant at high frequencies (46.7% vs. 8.3%), abnormal vestibular tests, abnormal oculocephalic response (13.3% vs. 0%), abnormal caloric test (26.7% vs. 0%) and abnormal computerized dynamic posturography with a predominant vestibular loss pattern (23.3% vs. 0%) frequencies were significantly higher in the PsA group than in the control group. No significant relationship was found between the presence of audiovestibular symptoms in patients with PsA and the specific patterns, diagnosis age and disease duration of PsA. This study was the first to show oculographic, vestibular, and postural abnormalities in addition to auditory impairment in psoriatic disease. These tests, which show the presence of hypofunction (canal paresis) of the inner ear, supported that the audiovestibular distortion observed in PsA is at the peripheral etiology and the inner ear damage is at the cochleovestibular peripheral level. It has also been suggested that chronic inflammation may be responsible for audiovestibular findings in patients with PsA [15].

Akdag et al. (2015) investigated hearing changes with audiometric and otoacoustic emission tests in the age-gender matched prospective case-control study involving 31 PsA patients. As a result of the study, statistically significant differences (especially at high frequencies) were observed between pure tone audiometry in all frequencies and right and left emission at the 4.0 and 1.0 Hz in PsA patients versus controls. No significant relationship was found between the duration of PsA and the severity of hearing loss. Except for right ear audio at 2000 Hz, no correlation was found between the PASI measurement of PsA severity and hearing loss. In addition, no significant relationship was found between PASI scores and the degree of hearing changes. These data showed to the authors that the degree of hearing change was not related to the severity of PsA symptoms. Overall, mean hearing thresholds and otoacoustic emissions were detected to be impaired in PsA patients. With these results, it was thought that the inner ear injury is due to cochlear chronic damage caused by disruption of the inner ear microcirculation rather than acute inflammatory reactivation of the disease [16].

Aydın et al.'s study (2015) did not find any hearing loss with pure tone audiometry and transient evoked autoacoustic emission measurements in 41 patients with mild and moderate psoriasis. Hearing thresholds in all frequencies with pure tone audiometry were detected higher in patients with psoriasis than controls. Although the excitability, response values and signal:noise ratios according to frequencies were lower in the transient evoked autoacoustic emission test compared to the controls, these differences were not statistically significant. In addition, a relationship was not demonstrated between PASI score and psoriasis duration and SNHL [17].

In 2016, a case-control study involving 24 PsA patients (younger than 60 years old) conducted by Gunes et al. demonstrated bilateral symmetrical SNHL in 3 patients within the PsA group. When hearing frequencies between 4000 and 6000 Hz and the distortion product otoacoustic emission values at 3000 and 4000 Hz were evaluated in the PsA group, statistically significant differences were found compared to the control group. This study demonstrating that inner ear functions have been affected in patients with PsA provides strong evidence that it is necessary to monitor these patients regarding SNHL, which may cause serious disability, in order to take precautions against the development of sudden deafness [18].

Hapa et al. (2016) found significant differences between patients with psoriasis and controls in terms of median pure tone averages variables in a case-control study involving 50 psoriasis patients. However, no significant differences were observed between median pure tone averages variables according to the distribution of the lesions, previous systemic medications, disease duration and PASI scores. Considering the hearing levels of patients with psoriasis according to certain hearing frequencies (500, 1000, 2000, 4000, 8000 and 16,000 Hz), a statistically significant difference was detected between patients with psoriasis and the control group. It was determined that all the frequencies which show statistical significance (the median of hearing level at frequencies 500–4000 Hz) were not lower than 20 decibels, but the hearing levels of patients with psoriasis at higher frequencies (such as 8000 and 16,000 Hz) were lower than 20 decibels. This result indicated to the authors that psoriasis patients have hearing loss at high frequencies [19].

Amor-Dorado et al.'s vestibular evaluation study (2017) involving 60 PsA patients observed that the frequencies of abnormal oculocephalic response (13.3% vs. 0%) and abnormal caloric test (26.7% vs. 0%) were found higher than the controls. The frequencies of abnormal clinical test of sensory integration and balance test with vestibular loss pattern (33% vs. 6%) and abnormal computerized dynamic posturography test (23.3% vs. 0%) also increased significantly in PsA patients, indicating that oculographic findings have been frequent in PsA [20].

Temel et al.'s study (2017) including 61 psoriasis patients detected significant differences between the patients and controls in terms of audiovestibular symptoms and the values of the audiometric tests (pure tone average, speech recognition threshold, speech discrimination). While psoriasis patients had higher speech reception threshold than the control group, the speech discrimination test was found to be lower levels. The mean bone conduction and air conduction hearing thresholds were observed to be higher for all frequencies in the patients. These differences were found to be statistically significant at high frequencies (2.4 and 6 kHz). According to audiograms, high frequency bilateral symmetrical SNHL was detected in psoriasis patients compared to the controls. Although the vestibular abnormalities in psoriasis patients were demonstrated to be more common than the control group, only saccadic test values were observed to be statistically significant. No significant relationship was found between the presence of audiovestibular abnormalities and clinical patterns of psoriasis, duration or severity of the disease, concomitant PsA, nail involvement or use of anti-psoriatic drugs [21].

In a case-control study involving 77 psoriatic patients of Borgia et al. (2018), tympanogram abnormalities and hearing loss detected in the psoriasis group were found to be significantly more frequent than the control group (52.6% vs. 14.9%). Most of them were shown to had SNHL (SNHL in 57 ears, conductive hearing loss in 9 ears, and mixed-type hearing loss in the remaining 15 ears). In terms of hearing loss, the difference between both groups was observed to be significant only for SNHL. The frequency of hearing loss, mostly of the sensorineural type, increased with age at a higher rate in the psoriatic patients. Hearing loss frequency was demonstrated to be higher in the patients with psoriasis duration >10 years (mainly of conductive and mixed type), metabolic syndrome, higher body mass index levels (overweight/obesity) or smoking habit. In patients with arthropathic psoriasis, conductive and mixed hearing loss were detected to be more common than non-arthropathic ones. In addition, it was observed that the patients with hearing loss had higher clinical severity of psoriasis determined by PASI and Dermatology Life Quality Index scores [22].

In a case-control study involving 29 psoriasis patients, Vir et al. (2019) found statistically significant differences between patients and controls for pure tone thresholds at high frequencies, and for distortion product otoacoustic emission responses and signal:noise ratio at all frequencies. According to these findings, it was reported that the outer hair cells damage of cochlea causes high-frequency hearing loss in psoriasis patients [23].

In a case-control study including 50 psoriasis patients of Gurel et al. (2019), both the left ear and right ear hearing threshold values at 2000 Hz and the right ear hearing threshold values at 4000 and 8000 Hz were significantly higher in the psoriasis group than the control group. It was detected that the values of the psoriasis group were statistically significantly higher in terms of both the left ear and right ear mean air conduction and bone conduction hearing thresholds. In the correlation analysis between PASI score or disease duration and hearing loss, no significant relationship was observed [24].

Finally, in a case-control study to evaluate the audiovestibular system in 32 psoriasis patients without joint involvement, Ertugrul et al. (2020) did not find any significant differences between the groups in terms of hearing test results (pure tone audiometry and distortion product otoacoustic emission). However, in balance tests, the abnormal caloric test response was detected to be significantly higher in the psoriatic patients. They also mentioned that the severity of psoriasis rather than its duration is more important for vestibular system. No significant association was found between the Fitzpatrick skin type, medical treatments, the onset age of or clinical pattern of psoriasis and audiovestibular findings [25].

3. Discussion

Since the immunological basis of psoriasis has been understood in recent years, it is emphasized that the disease is not limited to the skin but a T cell-mediated systemic disease with various chronic and progressive comorbidities [37–42]. Like other diseases in this group, many IMIDs can appear in association with psoriasis [39–41]. The chronology of IMIDs associated with psoriasis was investigated by Andersen et al. in a large-scale study (psoriasis patients = 10.923; general population controls = 109.230). It was observed that approximately 20% of the patients with psoriasis developed ≥1 IMID, this risk was about five times higher than the general population, and most IMIDs had been diagnosed before psoriasis except PsA [43]. Many studies have demonstrated that some major comorbidities including PsA (mainly associated), metabolic syndrome, diabetes mellitus, coronary heart disease, hyperlipidemia, hypertension, obesity, inflammatory bowel disease, uveitis, obstructive sleep apnea, non-alcoholic fatty liver disease and psychiatric disturbances are more frequent than the normal population as a result of chronic inflammation in patients with psoriasis. These observations indicate the necessity to investigate for possible morbidities that may accompany psoriasis [39–42]. In the IMPROVE (incentives for health care management based on patient-related outcomes and value) study conducted in Denmark, it was observed that psoriasis has had a significant impact on health care costs, income and employment. In addition, psoriasis was also associated with a range of comorbidities (with higher incidence of cardiovascular and psychiatric conditions) compared to controls [8]. In another study of Baviere et al., it was shown that 30.6% of patients with PsA had ≥3 comorbidities but the type of comorbidity had more effects than the number of comorbidities [9].

Immune-mediated or autoimmune SNHL may be a primary localized disease caused by region-specific immune-mediated damage in the inner ear or may be a secondary expression of a systemic autoimmune disease. It is characterized by bilateral, asymmetrical, often asynchronous and fluctuant deafness, which clinically worsens in weeks or months [29–31]. Tinnitus, dizziness and imbalance can also be accompanied [30]. Clinical diagnosis of autoimmune SNHL, mostly seen in women and middle age, can be confirmed with a positive response to steroid therapy following exclusion of other possible causes [31]. In SNHL accompanying autoimmune diseases, inner ear involvement has been observed to be more pronounced at high frequency hearing thresholds. Therefore, evaluating the high frequencies of the hearing values along with the conventional frequencies in patients who do not identify the clinical symptoms of hearing loss can help detect the presence of early hearing impairment and measures against sudden hearing loss can be taken [29–31, 44]. Extended high-frequency audiometry, expressing sounds above 8000 Hz, has been proven as a promising tool for the early detection of hearing disorders [18, 31]. In a population-based study using a National Health Insurance Service National Sample Cohort data from Korea, Jeong et al. investigated the risk of sudden SNHL (commonly known as sudden deafness; a SNHL of 30 dB or more over at least three contiguous audiometric frequencies occurring over less than 3 days) in patients with autoimmune diseases and compared these findings to a control group. As a result of this study, the risk of sudden SNHL was found significantly higher in the autoimmune-disease group than in the controls (autoimmune-disease group: 145/13.250 = 1.09%; control group: 484/6.250 = 0.73%) [45]. Due to unilateral involvement in most of the sudden SNHL cases, it may be difficult to demonstrate the relationship of this condition with an autoimmune disease. Therefore, it should not be ignored that immune-mediated SNHL can rarely occur with unilateral involvement in the initial period, similar to sudden SNHL [35, 36].

T lymphocyte-mediated cytotoxicity, vasculitis and immune complex accumulation have been generally accepted as the main causal mechanisms in development of SNHL accompanying immune-mediated diseases [29, 32]. Kumar et al. proposed a different theory like that "In autoimmune and chronic inflammatory diseases, prolonged serum levels of peripherally active T lymphocytes and proinflammatory cytokines (e.g., IL-1, IL-6, TNF-α) may cause degeneration in the cochlea, so hearing loss is a result of the harmful and unexpected effects of circulating inflammatory mediators". This model was recommended firstly based on patients with ulcerative colitis and was argued to be applicable for other chronic inflammatory and autoimmune diseases [46]. Although the cause of psoriasis disease is precisely unknown, recent genetic and immunological studies have shown that it is also a chronic IMID [38, 39]. Considering that the deteriorations in the structure and functions of the skin, nails and joints in psoriasis are primarily related to systemic chronic inflammation, it has been suggested that the same pathological process may have similar effects on the cochlea and play a role in the development of immune-mediated hearing loss [37, 47, 48]. T helper (Th) 1, Th17 and Th22 lymphocytes, which play a role in the pathogenesis of psoriasis, are active in psoriatic skin and circulation. The levels of proinflammatory cytokines (IL-1, IL-6, TNF-α, etc.) have also increased. It is well-known that TNF-α is an important mediator that also enhances the synthesis of other proinflammatory cytokines such as IL-1, IL-6, and IL-8 [3, 37]. The excellent response of psoriasis to TNF-α inhibitors has been emphasized that the role of TNF-α is indisputable in the pathogenesis of psoriasis [49]. Another situation demonstrating the effects of current cytokines on hearing loss is that TNF-α inhibitor drugs have been used successfully in the treatment of SNHL [50, 51]. Ertugrul et al. suggested that the immune response of the inner ear in psoriasis is likely to be impaired by antibody response in the endolymphatic sac, which has a central role in immunological activity within the inner ear and has capable of both processing antigen and producing antibodies [25]. In the case of inflammation in the body, accumulation of leukocytes entering the cochlea from the peripheral circulation and local immunoglobulin production cause an inflammatory reaction. This local inflammation leads to the degeneration of organ of corti, stria vascularis and spiral ganglion, which ultimately causes SNHL [32].

High frequency hearing loss in patients with psoriasis and PsA may be associated with chronic inflammation and autoimmune etiology [14, 15, 19, 21, 23]. It has been postulated that comorbidities such as metabolic syndrome and high body mass index values, which are frequently accompanied by psoriasis, may also contribute to hearing impairment [22]. Comorbid hypertension was determined as independent risk factor for sudden SNHL in psoriasis patients by Yen et al. [12]. In addition, it has been suggested that the correlation between high PASI scores and hearing loss at medium and high frequencies may be related to the increase of the mediators responsible for psoriatic disease to high levels in exacerbation periods [14, 22, 25]. However, in most studies, no relationship was found between the duration of psoriatic disease, clinical patterns of psoriasis, medical treatments and patient age, and hearing loss and/or audiovestibular dysfunction [14–17, 19, 21, 24, 25]. In studies demonstrating significant hearing loss in psoriasis patients, accompanying joint involvement was observed in 5.8% to 51.9% of them [14, 21, 22]. It has been mentioned that the presence of joint involvement in patients with psoriasis may lead to a more chronic inflammatory process and so adversely affect hearing [25]. Indeed, studies evaluating the hearing of psoriasis patients have different results, but it has been reported that hearing was adversely affected in all studies examining patients with PsA [15, 16, 18, 20]. It has been stated that PsA, which condition facilitates additional bone formation, can disrupt outer hair cell integrity through the formation of autoimmune-mediated fibro-osseous deposits in the cochlea [16].

The main treatment for autoimmune inner ear disease is by corticosteroids, and significant improvement of hearing impairment has also been reported in previous PsA cases following steroid administration [27–29]. Moreover, promising advances have been performed in the treatment of immune-mediated inner ear disease with various TNF-α inhibitors (etanercept, infliximab, golimumab; as used in other underlying autoimmune diseases or as form of local intratimpanic infusion), demonstrating them to be effective in reducing inflammation and hearing loss in cochlear diseases [44, 51]. Nonetheless, if hearing loss still occurs, cochlear implantation is a safe and effective method for the auditory rehabilitation of severe SNHL [44, 52]. However, flap complications are more common in cases such as psoriasis, where the risk of surgical site infection is higher than normal patients. It has been beneficial to add perioperative antipsoriatic topical agents and/or UVB phototherapy to standard infection prophylaxis in terms of reducing postoperative infection and sequelae [52].

4. Conclusion

The relationship between psoriasis/PsA and audiovestibular dysfunction supports the need for further studies aimed at better identification of the underlying pathogenic mechanisms, and accordingly to update diagnostic and even treatment approaches. It is well known by most dermatologists that psoriasis is a lifelong multisystemic chronic inflammatory disease rather than just a skin and/or joint condition. It should also be remembered that psoriatic disease, which has become the target of modern biological treatments today, is often accompanied by certain comorbidities such as metabolic syndrome, cardiovascular disease and obesity. For this reason, psoriasis and its associations should be approached in an integrated manner as well as related physicians should be in regular coordination with specialists in a special multidisciplinary team. However, it is obvious that physicians, especially dermatologists and rheumatologists, need to be more aware of the prevalence of hearing loss in psoriasis patients. It should be kept in mind that subclinical SNHL is a neglected but an important comorbidity in patients with psoriasis and PsA. Psoriatic patients, particularly with severe clinical symptoms, arthropathy, obesity, hypertension and metabolic syndrome, should be followed up with regular audiometric tests even if there is no subjective hearing complaint. In fact, regardless of clinical severity or type of psoriasis, evaluation of all psoriatic patients for the audiovestibular perspective would be more useful for the future quality of life of patients. If patients with psoriasis have any hearing problem, they should be addressed to otorhinolaryngologists and audiometrists in terms of the follow-up to possible development of audiovestibular dysfunction and sudden SNHL.

Author details

Sevgi Akarsu
Department of Dermatology, Faculty of Medicine, Dokuz Eylul University, Izmir, Turkey

*Address all correspondence to: sevgi.akarsu@deu.edu.tr

References

[1] Raychaudhuri SP. A cutting edge overview: psoriatic disease. Clin Rev Allergy Immunol. 2013;44:109-13. doi: 10.1007/s12016-012-8309-z.

[2] Kimmel GW, Lebwohl M. Psoriasis: overview and diagnosis. Evidence-Based Psoriasis. 2018:1-16. doi: 10.1007/978-3-319-90107-7-1.

[3] Chiricozzi A, Romanelli P, Volpe E, Borsellino G, Romanelli M. Scanning the immunopathogenesis of psoriasis. Int J Mol Sci. 2018;19:179. doi: 10.3390/ijms19010179.

[4] Liang Y, Sarkar MK, Tsoi LC, Gudjonsson JE. Psoriasis: a mixed autoimmune and autoinflammatory disease. Curr Opin Immunol. 2017;49:1-8. doi: 10.1016/j.coi.2017.07.007.

[5] Kovitwanichkanont T, Chong AH, Foley P. Beyond skin deep: addressing comorbidities in psoriasis. Med J Aust. 2020;212:528-534. doi: 10.5694/mja2.50591.

[6] Rizzello F, Olivieri I, Armuzzi A, Ayala F, Bettoli V, Bianchi L, Cimino L, Costanzo A, Cristaudo A, D'Angelo S, Daperno M, Fostini AC, Galeazzi M, Gilio M, Gionchetti P, Gisondi P, Lubrano E, Marchesoni A, Offidani A, Orlando A, Pugliese D, Salvarani C, Scarpa R, Vecchi M, Girolomoni G. Multidisciplinary management of spondyloarthritis-related immune-mediated inflammatory disease. Adv Ther. 2018;35:545-562. doi: 10.1007/s12325-018-0672-6.

[7] Mease PJ, Etzel CJ, Huster WJ, Muram TM, Armstrong AW, Lisse JR, Rebello S, Dodge R, Murage MJ, Greenberg JD, Malatestinic WN. Understanding the association between skin involvement and joint activity in patients with psoriatic arthritis: experience from the Corrona Registry. RMD Open. 2019;5:e000867. doi: 10.1136/rmdopen-2018-000867.

[8] Thomsen SF, Skov L, Dodge R, Hedegaard MS, Kjellberg J. Socioeconomic costs and health inequalities from psoriasis: a cohort study. Dermatology. 2019;235:372-379. doi: 10.1159/000499924.

[9] Bavière W, Deprez X, Houvenagel E, Philippe P, Deken V, Flipo RM, Paccou J. Association between comorbidities and quality of life in psoriatic arthritis: results from a multicentric cross-sectional study. J Rheumatol. 2020;47:369-376. doi: 10.3899/jrheum.181471.

[10] Wipperman J. Otitis externa. Prim Care. 2014;41:1-9. doi: 10.1016/j.pop.2013.10.001.

[11] Dopytalska K, Sobolewski P, Błaszczak A, Szymańska E, Walecka I. Psoriasis in special localizations. Reumatologia. 2018;56:392-398. doi: 10.5114/reum.2018.80718.

[12] Yen YC, Lin YS, Weng SF, Lai FJ. Risk of sudden sensorineural hearing loss in patients with psoriasis: a retrospective cohort study. Am J Clin Dermatol. 2015;16:213-220. doi: 10.1007/s40257-015-0117-9.

[13] Karabulut H, Karadag AS, Dagli M, Acar B, Babademez MA, Sahin Y, Karasen RM. Investigation of hearing and outer hair cell function of cochlea in patients with psoriasis. Int Adv Otol. 2010;6:239-244.

[14] Guvenc SC, Turan H, Yilmaz S, Yanik ME, Berada A, Aliagaoglu C. [Assesment of hearing loss in patients with psoriasis]. Turkderm. 2012;46:15-19.

[15] Amor-Dorado JC, Barreira-Fernandez MP, Pina T, Vázquez-Rodríguez TR, Llorca J, González-Gay MA. Investigations into audiovestibular manifestations

in patients with psoriatic arthritis. J Rheumatol. 2014;41:2018-2026. doi: 10.3899/jrheum.140559.

[16] Akdag M, Uçmak D, Özkurt FE, Bozkurt M, Akkurt ZM, Topçu İ. Evaluation of hearing and outer hair cell function of cochlea in patients with psoriatic arthritis. Clin Exp Otorhinolaryngol. 2015;8:183-188. doi: 10.3342/ceo.2015.8.3.183.

[17] Aydın E, Dogan B, Karabacak E, Karabudak Abuaf O, Erkul E, Saglam O, Dursun E. [Evaluation of hearing with audiometry and transient evoked otoacoustic emission in patients with mild and moderate psoriasis]. Gulhane Medical Journal. 2015;57:98-101. doi: 10.5455/gulhane.178662

[18] Gunes A, Gundogdu I, Mutlu M, Ozturk EA, Cakci A, Akin I. Functions of the inner ear in psoriatic arthritis. Auris Nasus Larynx. 2016;43:626-631. doi: 10.1016/j.anl.2016.02.004.

[19] Hapa A, Suslu N, Karaduman A, Budak B, Ersoy Evans S, Sennaroglu L. Evaluation of hearing in patients with psoriasis considering the disease severity. ENT Updates. 2016;6:140-144. doi:10.2399/jmu.2016003006.

[20] Amor-Dorado JC, Barreira-Fernandez MP, Llorca J, González-Gay MA. Oculographic, clinical test of sensory integration and balance and computerized dynamic Posturography findings in patients with psoriatic arthritis. Otol Neurotol. 2017;38:448-453.doi: 10.1097/MAO.0000000000001296.

[21] Temel IC, Bilgic TA, Alpsoy E, Yılmaz E, Akman Karakas A, Bozkurt S, Agirdir BV. Evaluations of audiovestibular manifestations in patients with psoriasis. Turk J Dermatol. 2017;11:162-167. doi: 10.4274/tdd.3307.

[22] Borgia F, Ciodaro F, Guarneri F, Bartolotta A, Papaianni V, Guarneri C, Catalano N, Galletti F, Cannavò SP. Auditory system involvement in psoriasis. Acta Derm Venereol. 2018;98:655-659. doi: 10.2340/00015555-2937.

[23] Vir D, Sharma P, Mahajan R, Dogra S, Bakshi J, Panda NK. Investigation of high-frequency hearing loss and outer hair cell function of the cochlea in patients with psoriasis: a case-control study. Clin Exp Dermatol. 2019;44:520-523. doi: 10.1111/ced.13805.

[24] Gurel G, Kantekin Y, Haberal Can I. Do patients with psoriasis suffer from hearing loss? Turkiye Klinikleri J Dermatol. 2019;29:101-107. doi: 10.5336/dermato.*2019*-70659.

[25] Ertugrul G, Ertugrul S, Soylemez E. Evaluation of audiovestibular system in psoriasis patients without joint involvement. Dermatol Ther. 2020:e13396. doi: 10.1111/dth.13396.

[26] Maune S, Frese KA, Mrowietz U, Reker U. Toxic inner ear damage in topical treatment of psoriasis with salicylates. Laryngorhinootologie. 1997;76:368-370.

[27] Srikumar S, Deepak MK, Basu S, Kumar BN. Sensorineural hearing loss associated with psoriatic arthritis. J Laryngol Otol. 2004;118:909-11. doi: 10.1258/0022215042703813.

[28] Giani T, Simonini G, Lunardi C, Puccetti A, De Martino M, Falcini F. Juvenile psoriatic arthritis and acquired sensorineural hearing loss in a teenager: is there an association? Clin Exp Rheumatol. 2006;24:344-346.

[29] Mijovic T, Zeitouni A, Colmegna I. Autoimmune sensorineural hearing loss: the otology–rheumatology interface. Rheumatology (Oxford). 2013;52:780-789. doi:10.1093/rheumatology/ket009.

[30] Ralli M, D'Aguanno V, Di Stadio A, De Virgilio A, Croce A, Longo L, Greco A, de Vincentiis M.

Audiovestibular symptoms in systemic autoimmune diseases. J Immunol Res. 2018;2018:5798103. doi: 10.1155/2018/5798103.

[31] Isaacson JE, Vora NM. Differential diagnosis and treatment of hearing loss. Am Fam Physician 2003; 68: 1125-1132.

[32] Berrocal JR, Ramírez-Camacho R. Sudden sensorineural hearing loss: supporting the immunologic theory. Ann Otol Rhinol Laryngol. 2002;111:989-997. doi: 10.1177/000348940211101107.

[33] Lehnhardt E. [Sudden Hearing Disorders Occurring Simultaneously or Successively on Both Sides]. Z Laryngol Rhinol Otol. 1958;37:1-16.

[34] McCabe BF. Autoimmune sensorineural hearing loss. Ann Otol Rhinol Laryngol. 1979;88:585-589.

[35] Young YH. Contemporary review of the causes and differential diagnosis of sudden sensorineural hearing loss. Int J Audiol. 2020;59:243-253. doi: 10.1080/14992027.2019.1689432.

[36] Rossini BAA, Penido NO, Munhoz MSL, Bogaz EA, Curi RS. Sudden sensorioneural hearing loss and autoimmune systemic diseases. Int Arch Otorhinolaryngol. 2017;21:213-223. doi: 10.1055/s-0036-1586162.

[37] Grän F, Kerstan A, Serfling E, Goebeler M, Muhammad K. Current developments in the immunology of psoriasis. Yale J Biol Med. 2020;93:97-110.

[38] Ayala-Fontánez N, Soler DC, McCormick TS. Current knowledge on psoriasis and autoimmune diseases. Psoriasis (Auckl). 2016;6:7-32. doi: 10.2147/PTT.S64950.

[39] Furue K, Ito T, Tsuji G, Kadono T, Nakahara T, Furue M. Autoimmunity and autoimmune co-morbidities in psoriasis. Immunology. 2018;154:21-27. doi: 10.1111/imm.12891.

[40] Sundarrajan S, Arumugam M. Comorbidities of psoriasis - Exploring the links by network approach. PLoS One. 2016;11:e0149175. doi: 10.1371/journal.pone.0149175.

[41] Korman NJ. Management of psoriasis as a systemic disease: what is the evidence? Br J Dermatol. 2020;182:840-848. doi: 10.1111/bjd.18245.

[42] Oliveira Mde F, Rocha Bde O, Duarte GV. Psoriasis: classical and emerging comorbidities. An Bras Dermatol. 2015;90:9-20. doi: 10.1590/abd1806-4841.20153038.

[43] Andersen YMF, Wu JJ, Thyssen JP, Egeberg A. Chronologic order of appearance of immune-mediated inflammatory diseases relative to diagnosis of psoriasis. J Am Acad Dermatol. 2019;81:1283-1291. doi:10.1016/j.jaad.2019.04.033

[44] Sakano H, Harris JP. Emerging options in immune-mediated hearing loss. Laryngoscope Investig Otolaryngol. 2018;4:102-108. doi: 10.1002/lio2.205.

[45] Jeong J, Lim H, Lee K, Hong CE, Choi HS. High risk of sudden sensorineural hearing loss in several autoimmune diseases according to a population-based National Sample Cohort Study. Audiol Neurootol. 2019;24:224-230. doi: 10.1159/000502677.

[46] Kumar BN, Walsh RM, Wilson PS, Carlin WV. Sensorineural hearing loss and ulcerative colitis. J Laryngol Otol. 1997;111:277-278.

[47] Cannavò SP, Guarneri F, Giuffrida R, Aragona E, Guarneri C. Evaluation of cutaneous surface parameters in psoriatic patients. Skin Res Technol. 2017;23:41-47. doi: 10.1111/srt.12299.

[48] Yoon SH, Kim ME, Kim HY, Lee JS, Jang CH. Inflammatory cytokines and mononuclear cells in sudden sensorineural hearing loss. J Laryngol Otol. 2019;133:95-101. doi: 10.1017/S0022215119000100.

[49] Wcisło-Dziadecka D, Zbiciak-Nylec M, Brzezińska-Wcisło L, Mazurek U. TNF-α in a molecularly targeted therapy of psoriasis and psoriatic arthritis. Postgrad Med J. 2016;92(1085):172-178. doi: 10.1136/postgradmedj-2015-133419.

[50] Wang X, Truong T, Billings PB, Harris JP, Keithley EM. Blockage of immune-mediated inner ear damage by etanercept. Otol Neurotol. 2003;24:52-57. doi: 10.1097/00129492-200301000-00012.

[51] Rodrigues JC, Bachi ALL, Silva GAV, Rossi M, do Amaral JB, Lezirovitz K, de Brito R. New insights on the effect of TNF alpha blockade by gene silencing in noise-induced hearing loss. Int J Mol Sci. 2020;21:E2692. doi: 10.3390/ijms21082692.

[52] Basavaraj S, Wardrop P, Sivaji N, Shanks M, Allen AA. Cochlear implantation in psoriasis patients. Auris Nasus Larynx. 2007;34:221-223. doi: 10.1016/j.anl.2006.07.004.

Chapter 6

Enkephalin Therapy Improves Relapsing-Remitting Multiple Sclerosis

Chirag L. Patel, Ian S. Zagon, Gary A. Thomas and Patricia J. McLaughlin

Abstract

Multiple sclerosis (MS) is accompanied by decreases in serum endogenous enkephalin/endorphins and alterations in inflammatory cytokines. This retrospective analysis of serum levels was conducted in 53 patients with established relapsing-remitting MS treated with the disease-modifying therapies (DMT) glatiramer acetate, dimethyl fumarate or with the biotherapeutic low dose naltrexone (LDN) to elevate enkephalins, an off-label alternative. Opioid growth factor (OGF), an inhibitory endogenous opioid involved in modulating cellular replication, was measured and correlated to serum β-endorphin, IL-17A and TNFα. Results revealed that MS leads to a significant reduction in OGF levels in subjects on DMTs, but patients on LDN had OGF levels comparable to non-MS controls. Individuals on DMTs had significantly elevated TNFα levels, while IL-17A levels were significantly elevated only in patients taking dimethyl fumarate. A direct correlation was established between OGF and IL17A indicating a potential interaction between the OGF-OGFr axis and pro-inflammatory T-helper cells providing insight into the disease etiology.

Keywords: relapsing-remitting multiple sclerosis, serum cytokines, opioid growth factor, low-dose naltrexone, biomarkers

1. Introduction

Multiple sclerosis (MS) is a demyelinating disorder with an underlying neuroinflammatory disease process affecting approximately 2.5 million people worldwide [1]. Traditionally, the disease has a greater prevalence in locations which are geographically north of the equator. In a study from 2015, North America and Europe had an average prevalence of greater than 100/100,000 individuals, whereas East Asia and Sub-Saharan Africa had rates of 2/100,000 individuals [2].

1.1 Environmental and genetic risk factors

To better understand this disparity, an umbrella systemic review looked at the possible environmental risk factors involved in the development of multiple sclerosis [3]. An analysis of 44 potential risk factors was filtered down to 3 which were found to be profoundly significant: anti-Epstein-Barr Virus Nuclear Antigen IgG seropositivity, infectious mononucleosis, and smoking [3]. The hypothesis behind anti-EBVNA IgG suggests that late adolescence exposure to EBV leads to infectious mononucleosis with significantly elevated IgG titers when compared to individuals who were exposed at a younger age [4, 5]. These titers in turn correlate to an increased risk of developing multiple sclerosis. One study done on this, "high-hygiene" population found that individuals of the same age who were not infected with EBV had a 10-fold lower risk of developing multiple sclerosis when compared to their EBV infected counterparts [4]. The pathology linking EBV titers to the initiation of multiple sclerosis are not yet clear, however it may increase the risk for an autoimmune type response as was seen with Systemic Lupus Erythematous and EBV [4, 6].

Several studies have shown a direct correlation between cigarette smoking and incidence of multiple sclerosis [4, 7–10]. There is some variability in the literature between gender and age groups. One study suggests cigarette smoking at a younger age (<26.4 years) is associated with a 50% increased risk that was alleviated in individuals who were older [8]. A Canadian study comparing gender and smoking history and found that 71.5% males diagnosed with multiple sclerosis had previously smoked compared to 63.6% of females [10]. Smoking has previously been defined in several pathologies including cancer, asthma, atherosclerosis and heart disease, but within multiple sclerosis, the mechanism is still not understood.

Genetic risk factors have come to the forefront of current research as some have been linked with modulation of the immune response. Initial studies linked loci of the Major Histocompatibility Complex (MHC) and Human Leukocyte Antigen (HLA) as contributing risk in the development and progression of multiple sclerosis [4, 11–14]. In particular, HLA-*DRB1 and DQB1* gene loci were thought to play a role in developing the inherent autoimmunity associated with the disease [11, 14–16].

1.2 Diagnosis of multiple sclerosis

In 2001, the McDonald criteria were created to streamline the diagnosis of multiple sclerosis even with its heterogeneous clinical presentation. The initial criteria introduced the utility of magnetic resonance imaging (MRI) and integration of multiple clinical symptoms while removing "clinically definite" and "possible multiple sclerosis" as alternatives [17]. Since 2001, 3 additional revisions have been made to the initial McDonald criteria: 2005, 2010 and 2017 [18–21]. Diagnosis of multiple sclerosis is now approached based on dissemination of time (temporal) and space. Dissemination in space is defined by either clinical presentation or MRI. Clinically, an individual must have symptoms which are distinct to different anatomical locations of the central nervous system. Usually, individuals present with optic neuritis or ocular symptoms and later acquire gait disturbances or peripheral weakness [18, 22]. On MRI, dissemination in space requires T2 evident lesions located in at least two distinct zones such as periventricular, infratentorial, juxtacortical or within the spinal cord [18, 22]. Dissemination in time requires the presence of a gadolinium-enhancing lesion on MRI, indicating an acute or active lesion, along with a non-enhancing lesion [18, 22]. The presence of a new lesion alone can meet the criteria if it is performed on a follow up scan. Essentially, dissemination in time seeks to distinguish multiple sclerosis symptomatology both typical and atypical from other neurological disorders which may share certain characteristics. As of McDonald 2010, CSF analysis is not required in order to make a definitive diagnosis [19–22]. Analysis of CSF typically presents with mildly elevated white blood cell count, protein, and IgG oligoclonal bands which are not typically seen in serum analysis [22]. IgG oligoclonal bands can be found in 90% of multiple sclerosis patients, but it may have a greater role in distinguishing individuals with clinically isolated syndrome (CIS) [20]. Some studies demonstrated that CSF oligoclonal bands increase the specificity of MR imaging in adults with CIS and pediatrics with radiologically isolated syndrome (RIS) [23, 24]. Beyond the diagnosis of multiple sclerosis, CSF analysis may help distinguish other immune mediated neurological and non-neurological pathologies.

1.3 Clinical presentation of multiple sclerosis

The disease course of multiple sclerosis is usually defined into four clinical subtypes: clinically isolated syndrome (CIS), relapsing-remitting multiple sclerosis, secondary progressive multiple sclerosis, and primary progressive multiple sclerosis. A majority of patients have a disease course defined by stages of relapses and remission which may later translate into the secondary progressive form [25]. Clinically, relapses are defined as distinct episodes of neurological dysfunction which can present as a wide array of symptoms including sensory defects of the limbs, visual loss, motor defects, gait disturbances, vertigo, heat sensitivity (Uhthoff phenomenon), Lhermitte sign and fatigue [22, 26]. However, multiple sclerosis can present atypically in younger individuals, making it difficult to diagnosis properly. The initial episodes are followed by periods of remission where the patient will fully or partially regain normal function and be deemed neurologically stable [27]. In the long term, as some individuals transition from the relapsing-remitting form to secondary progressive, relapses no longer occur, yet patients will experience worsening neurological function [27]. After 10 years of disease, 50% of individuals with relapsing-remitting multiple sclerosis will convert to secondary-progressive, whereas after 25 years of the disorder, more than 90% of the individuals have secondary progressive multiple sclerosis [14].

Prior to establishing criteria for dissemination in time and space, individuals may present with clinically isolated syndrome (CIS) or radiologically isolated syndrome (RIS). Clinically isolated syndrome is defined as a clinical episode resembling a multiple sclerosis attack, after which there is full or partial recovery of neurological function [14, 20, 27]. Studies have shown that individuals with CIS may have an increased rate of conversion to multiple sclerosis especially with the presence of CSF oligoclonal bands and gadolinium enhancing lesions on MRI [14, 18, 20]. Incidental findings of cerebral and spinal cord plaques without a clinical phenotype are defined as radiologically isolated syndrome (RIS). In a 5-year study of 451 patients with RIS, 34% of individuals developed a clinical event for which 9.6% were defined as primary progressive multiple sclerosis [28]. Interestingly, this study was able to strongly correlate the presence of cervical or thoracic spinal cord lesions with the first clinical event [28]. With this increase risk of progression to multiple sclerosis, the utility of disease-modifying therapies and longitudinal monitoring of CIS and RIS has become a priority for clinicians.

1.4 Inflammation in multiple sclerosis

The direct cause of multiple sclerosis still eludes the scientific community; however, several hypotheses have emerged which have been utilized to develop disease-modifying therapies (DMTs) and alter the course of disease. Traditionally, multiple sclerosis has been considered a demyelinating disease of the white matter tracts leading to peripheral symptomatology with an underlying autoimmune cause. Recently, demyelination located in the cerebral cortex and deep gray matter has emerged as a marker of progressing neurological disability [13, 29, 30]. Damage seen to the CNS with infiltration of immune cells suggests the role of peripheral immune response leading to damage of the blood brain barrier prior to established demyelination. Peripheral inflammation in this case may be a result of a foreign pathogen (virus), autoimmune activation, or a combination of multiple events. Malpass [31] characterized the term "outside-in" based on evidence of cortical inflammation originating in the subarachnoid space in multiple sclerosis patients which transitioned into the white matter [32]. This further strengthens the argument for modulation of the peripheral inflammatory response which is facilitating early multiple sclerosis disease through activation of CD4 T lymphocytes. Once within the CNS, regional activation of microglia, astrocytes and macrophages occurs through expression of cytokines and chemokines from infiltration of T lymphocytes [13, 29, 30, 33]. Activation of specific subsets of CD4 lymphocytes dictates which cytokines are released. Pro-inflammatory cytokines are expressed after direct activation of Th1 and Th17 cells, whereas anti-inflammatory cytokines are a product of Th2 and T-regulatory cells [34–36]. Histopathology of the CNS white matter plaques has shown an abundance of macrophages, CD8, CD4 T lymphocytes, and B lymphocytes [13, 29, 30, 35]. Over time, the prolonged inflammation and infiltration of T and B lymphocytes leads to a disruption of the axonal-glial interaction which results in an increase in gray matter atrophy and axonal loss with marked demyelination [13, 29]. During the remission phase following each flare, there is some evidence to suggest a possible role for regulatory T cells with the induction of Foxp3 [37]. It is possible that during remission, a baseline level of inflammation is present; however, the expression of specific phenotypes of T lymphocytes shifts toward anti-inflammatory/regulatory rather than pro-inflammatory mechanisms. Based on these observations, vitamin D has emerged as a potential homeopathic regulator of immune cell function [2, 3, 38].

1.5 Current disease-modifying therapies

Currently, there is no definitive treatment for multiple sclerosis. Most approved therapies are focused on controlling peripheral inflammation and preventing migration across the blood brain barrier thereby reducing the incidence of acute flares [13, 30, 39, 40]. A majority of these therapies are administered orally, as an injection or through an infusion. With both invasive and non-invasive methods, side effects include increases in liver enzymes, injection site reactions, nausea, diarrhea, and most importantly, progressive multifocal leukoencephalopathy (PML) [39]. The primary therapies prescribed at our institution are Copaxone®, Gilenya®, and Tecfidera®. Copaxone®, glatiramer acetate is an immunomodulator that is FDA approved to reduce the frequency of relapses. Gilenya®, fingolimod, is also an immunomodulator that targets reduction in the number of relapses more than progression of disease. Tecfidera®, dimethyl fumarate, is a combination of fumaric acid esters that was originally approved for oral treatment of psoriasis. Because of the inconsistent or incomplete outcomes from treatment, as well as the evolving nature of the disorder, other biotherapies have been used as adjuvants.

1.6 Enkephalins as therapeutic treatment

One alternative biotherapeutic is the use of low doses of naltrexone (LDN), an opioid receptor antagonist. LDN is often used as an adjuvant to disease-modifying therapy to target fatigue associated with either the disorder or the medication. LDN has a strong profile of safety and tolerability [41–44]. Pilot studies utilizing LDN demonstrated that MS patients had an improvement in peripheral spasticity and mental health composite scores without inducing any side effects [42, 45]. In a retrospective analysis which compared LDN patients with LDN plus Copaxone® patients, there was no significant difference between the groups with respect to MRI, complete blood count, liver enzymes and the 25-foot walk test [44].

A number of published studies, clinical trials and anecdotal stories have supported the use of LDN as a beneficial therapy for multiple sclerosis [41–48]. The mechanism of action for this general antagonist is to block the interaction of Opioid Growth Factor (OGF) (chemically termed [Met^5]-enkephalin) from interacting at the nuclear-associated receptor OGFr. In addition to being a neurotransmitter, OGF is an inhibitory growth factor that suppresses proliferation of cells, including T and B cells associated with autoimmune disorders. Naltrexone was initially developed to treat opioid use disorder and alcoholism at a dosing of 50 mg where it acts as an opioid receptor antagonist for mu, delta, and kappa opiate receptors. At a dosage less than 5 mg, LDN acts as a biotherapeutic and modulates the activity of endogenous enkephalins and endorphins [49, 50]. In the multiple sclerosis patient population, endogenous [Met^5]-enkephalin (i.e., OGF) is reduced when compared to non-multiple sclerosis patients [51]. It is hypothesized that the reduction in serum levels of this inhibitory growth factor are unable to control the increase in T cell proliferation that occurs with immune-related flares. These T cells are the source of other pro-inflammatory cytokines that exacerbate the symptomatology of multiple sclerosis. The decreased serum levels of OGF appear to be compensated by low dosages of naltrexone (LDN).

1.6.1 Laboratory studies on LDN

Animal studies have been used to study both the mechanisms of LDN, as well as to establish the role of LDN as a biotherapy in mice with experimental autoimmune encephalomyelitis, an animal model of multiple sclerosis. In these studies, mice were immunized with antigens against myelin proteins—either myelin oligodendrocyte glycoprotein 35–55 or proteolipid peptides 139–151. The key component in the mechanistic pathway is the duration of opioid receptor blockade. This work is detailed in animal studies [51–57]. LDN produces an intermittent blockade of OGFr preventing OGF from binding and thereby increasing cellular replication, similar to what is seen with high doses of Naltrexone (HDN) through a prolonged blockade of OGFr [49]. Conversely, after the blockade has subsided, within 4–6 h, there is over proliferation of endogenous OGF and OGFr and a resulting exaggerated expression of p16 and p21 leading to promotion of cellular senescence [49].

A newly discovered pathway involves the antagonism of Toll-like receptor 4 (TLR4) by LDN as means to reduce neuroinflammation or persistent pain [58, 59]. Specifically, activation of Toll-like receptor 4 (TLR4) initiates the release of inflammatory cytokines: interleukin 1 (IL-1), tumor necrosis factor α (TNFα), nitric oxide (NO), and interferon β (IFNβ) [48, 60]. Currently, the relationship of the Toll-like receptor pathway to pro-inflammatory cytokine activation is not completely understood.

1.6.2 Clinical studies on LDN

Several studies have been conducted to evaluate multiple sclerosis patients who are prescribed LDN. The use of enkephalins, particularly OGF, has been demonstrated to be safe and tolerable in Phase I and Phase II studies of pancreatic cancer [61, 62]. LDN is widely used for treatment of other autoimmune disorders including Crohn's disease [63] and fibromyalgia [64].

1.6.3 Clinical studies on LDN and multiple sclerosis

Clinical trials using LDN for multiple sclerosis were conducted more than a decade ago, and most likely because it is widely used with no side-effects, government agencies are reluctant to support new trials. Three clinical trials have suggested that LDN increased the quality of life of patients with relapse-remitting or secondary progressive multiple sclerosis, without serious adverse effects [42, 43, 45]. Two retrospective studies examining charts of patients prescribed LDN alone, as well as in combination with the disease-modifying therapy Copaxone®, revealed no exacerbation of the disease or any substantial side effect for patients in either cohort [44]. In this study, the average length of disease was 14 years, with an average of 3 years on LDN alone. Clinical laboratory data revealed that patients on LDN alone had no significant differences in their blood chemistry, nutrition or liver data from patients on disease-modifying therapies.

However, these studies did not measure serum enkephalins, endorphins, or cytokines in an effort to gain more information on the mechanism of action for this biotherapeutic. A small study obtained stored serum from relapsing-remitting multiple sclerosis subjects and reported that enkephalin (i.e., OGF) levels were depressed relative to controls [51]. In the few individuals on LDN alone, serum OGF levels were elevated 2-fold in comparison to multiple sclerosis subjects on Copaxone® alone, suggesting that LDN may be effective at restoring serum enkephalin. Given this information, studies on both the mouse model of EAE and multiple sclerosis have been pursued to evaluate select cytokines that may be dysregulated in multiple sclerosis and possibly modulated by LDN (and enkephalin levels) and restored to normal levels.

2. Clinical study: enkephalin regulation of IL-17 in multiple sclerosis

A retrospective clinical study was designed to examine serum levels of cytokines and endogenous peptides, including [Met^5]-enkephalin.

2.1 Methods

Patients were identified through the Institute of Personalized Medicine at the Pennsylvania State University College of Medicine and had a clinically definitive diagnosis of relapsing–remitting multiple sclerosis [17, 18, 21, 36]. Selected individuals were between 18 and 70 years of age, of which 17 were males and 36 were females. Cohorts were established based on the disease-modifying therapy each of these patients was receiving. The five groups included multiple sclerosis patients receiving dimethyl fumarate, glatiramer acetate, low-dose naltrexone, or no disease-modifying therapy and a control group of non-multiple sclerosis patients. The 13 non-multiple sclerosis patients were recruited from the Neuroscience Institute and were age and gender matched to the study population. All patients were de-identified to the study team.

Blood was collected and stored in non-heparinized ethylenediaminetetraacetic acid (EDTA) tubes to prevent formation of a clot [65, 66]. Whole blood was centrifuged at 4°C for 10 min at 2500 rpm [65, 66]. Serum was aliquoted and stored long term at −80°C in 200 μL vials to prevent repeated freeze and thaw cycles.

Serum was analyzed using commercially produced sandwich or competitive enzyme labeled immunosorbent assay (ELISA). Opioid growth factor (MBS990622), β-endorphin (MBS770600), IL17A (MBS00565) and IL17 (MBS772095) ELISA kits were manufactured by MyBioSource (San Diego, CA); whereas the TNFα ELISA kit (EK0525) was purchased from BosterBio (Pleasanton, CA). Assays were completed following the manufacturer's recommendations; all samples and standards were run in duplicate and averaged for the data analyses. Chemiluminescence was measured using a BioTek microplate spectrophotometer and Gen5 software at 450 nm.

To ensure redundancy and reproducibility, duplicate samples were run on multiple ELISA kits from the same manufacturer.

Data analysis was performed using GraphPad Prism 8.0 software. Parametric data were analyzed using one-way analysis of variance (ANOVA) with post-hoc comparisons made using Newman-Keuls. Correlations were determined using Pearson's Correlation Coefficient (R). Significance was determined with a p value less than 0.05.

2.2 Results

A cohort of 53 patients was analyzed in this study, 40 of whom were individuals with an established diagnosis of relapsing-remitting (RR) multiple sclerosis and 13 who did not have multiple sclerosis. Patients with multiple sclerosis who received no disease-modifying therapy were designated as controls along with the 13 individuals with no diagnosis of multiple sclerosis. Within the control population, 17 were females and 7 males, whereas the study population had 19 females and 10 males. The age distribution between the cohorts of patients on treatment ranged between 25 and 69 years of age while the control cohort ranged in age from 25 to 78 years. Length of disease in the multiple sclerosis patient group was similar between the no-drug, dimethyl fumarate and LDN group which had mean lengths of 14.3, 10.4 and 16.5 years, respectively.

Serum OGF levels differed substantially between multiple sclerosis patients who declined therapy and control subjects considered non-multiple sclerosis (**Figure 1A**). OGF levels were more than three-fold higher in non-multiple sclerosis cohort relative to the no-drug cohort (93 ± 26 pg/ml). Because there is no diagnosis provided for the no-drug volunteers, it is difficult to more fully assess these data. Mean serum levels for RR-multiple sclerosis subjects prescribed disease-modifying therapy were comparable to serum values for the no-drug cohort, and significantly less than serum values for the non-multiple sclerosis cohort (**Figure 1B**). RR-multiple sclerosis patients receiving dimethyl fumarate had serum OGF values of 125 ± 22 pg/ml whereas those individuals receiving glatiramer acetate had serum levels of 136 ± 30 pg/ml. RR-multiple sclerosis subjects receiving LDN had mean OGF serum levels of 217 ± 29 mg/ml; these values did not differ from the non-multiple sclerosis cohort. Correlations between serum OGF levels and age or length of disease for cohorts of no drug, DMTs, or LDN are presented in **Figure 2A** and **B**, respectively. The association between age and serum OGF had an overall significance, with dimethyl fumarate subjects revealing a corresponding decrease in OGF serum values with increasing age ($p = 0.03$). Regarding the length of disease, RR-multiple sclerosis subjects taking LDN had comparable OGF serum values irrespective of having disease for 2 months or 33 years (**Figure 2B**). RR-multiple sclerosis subjects not taking any drugs (no-drug cohort) also displayed a biphasic response, suggesting that length of disease does not impact OGF serum. Analyses of OGF serum values by gender indicated that females had a pattern similar to that in **Figure 1B**. A majority of the males in this study received dimethyl fumarate and had serum OGF levels that ranged from 25 to 200 pg/ml; the small number of male subjects in the other cohorts prevented data analyses.

Serum β-endorphin levels were also measured in three cohorts of RR-multiple sclerosis subjects and non-multiple sclerosis subjects. Levels of serum β-endorphin ranged between ~1 ng/ml (no-drug and dimethyl fumarate cohorts) to the mean of 2.3 ng/ml (non-multiple sclerosis cohorts); individual samples ranged as high as 4 ng/ml in the non-multiple sclerosis cohort. Despite the variation, significant two-fold increases were recorded for non-multiple sclerosis and glatiramer acetate cohorts relative to no drug and dimethyl fumarate RR-multiple sclerosis

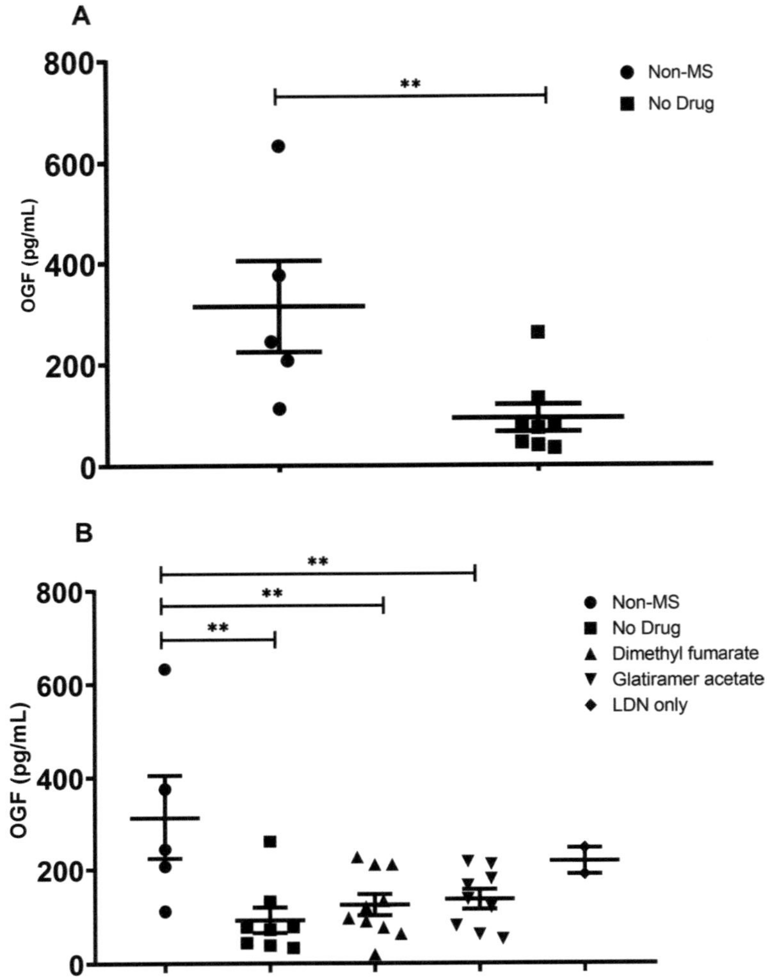

Figure 1.
Scatterplots of serum OGF levels (pg/ml) in (A) control subjects who were either non-multiple sclerosis subjects or (B) RR-MS patients who were not receiving any therapy (no drug) or RR-multiple sclerosis patients receiving dimethyl fumarate, glatiramer acetate, or low dose naltrexone (LDN). One-way ANOVA or t-tests were used to show the differences between groups. Significantly different from non-multiple sclerosis values at $p < 0.01$ *(**).*

individuals. Associations between age and β-endorphin revealed that endorphin levels were relatively stable within the population of RR-multiple sclerosis subjects on DMT.

With regard to serum levels of inflammatory cytokines, expression levels of two cytokines in serum are presented in **Figure 3**. Serum levels of IL-17 (A) and TNFα (B) were measured in RR-multiple sclerosis subjects on DMTs, LDN, or no-drug, as well as non-multiple sclerosis controls. Mean IL-17A (not shown) concentrations ranged from 27 ± 3 pg/ml (dimethyl fumarate) to 39 ± 10 pg/ml (glatiramer acetate group). Only one sample of blood from RR-multiple sclerosis patients on LDN was assayed; serum IL-17A value was 46 pg/ml. No differences in serum levels were noted between any therapeutic treatment and controls. IL-17 levels ranged from the mean 0.12 ng/ml recorded for non-multiple sclerosis cohort to 0.92 ± 0.35 ng/ml for the dimethyl fumarate group (**Figure 3A**); levels of the IL-17 cytokine recorded for these subjects differed significantly from glatiramer acetate and no-drug cohorts. RR-multiple sclerosis patients had a mean IL-17 cytokine level of near 0, whereas some individuals using dimethyl fumarate had more than 3 pg/ml IL-17 levels.

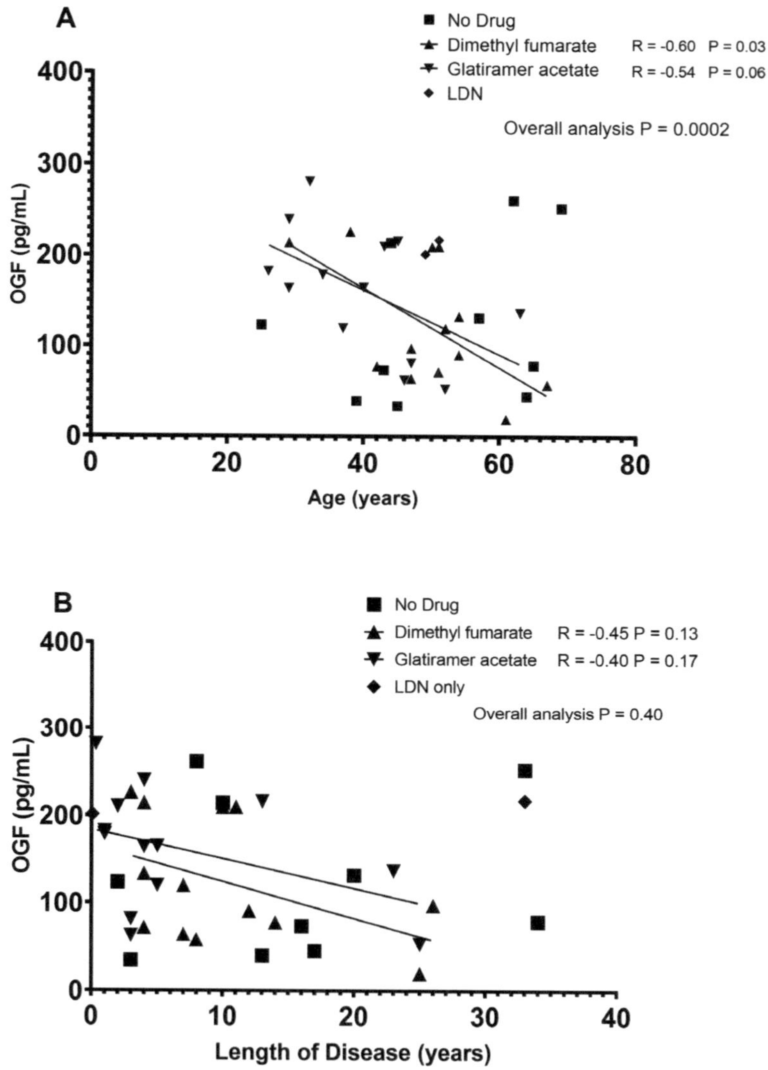

Figure 2.
Expression levels of serum OGF (pg/ml) measured by ELISA as a function of the age (years) of subject (A) or the length of disease (years) (B). Correlations were determined by Pearson's Correlation Coefficient (R) tests. P values less than 0.05 were considered significant.

Non-multiple sclerosis and RR-multiple sclerosis patients not taking any DMT had comparable TNFα values (16 ± 10 and 22 ± 3 pg/ml, respectively) (**Figure 3B**). RR-multiple sclerosis cohorts on DMTs had TNFα serum values that were at least 6-fold higher and differed significantly from the non-multiple sclerosis levels. Correlation analyses indicated that OGF (**Figure 4A**) and IL-17A (**Figure 4B**) were positively associated (R = 0.82), whereas TNFα values did not correlate (R = 0.20) with OGF serum values.

2.3 Discussion and summary

Cohorts of RR-multiple sclerosis patients on disease-modifying therapy, as well as a group of individuals diagnosed with RR-multiple sclerosis and taking LDN only were compared with control volunteers. in an assessment of peripheral serum levels of two endogenous neuropeptides—OGF (chemically termed methionine enkephalin) and β-endorphin, as well as 3 cytokines that are known to be involved

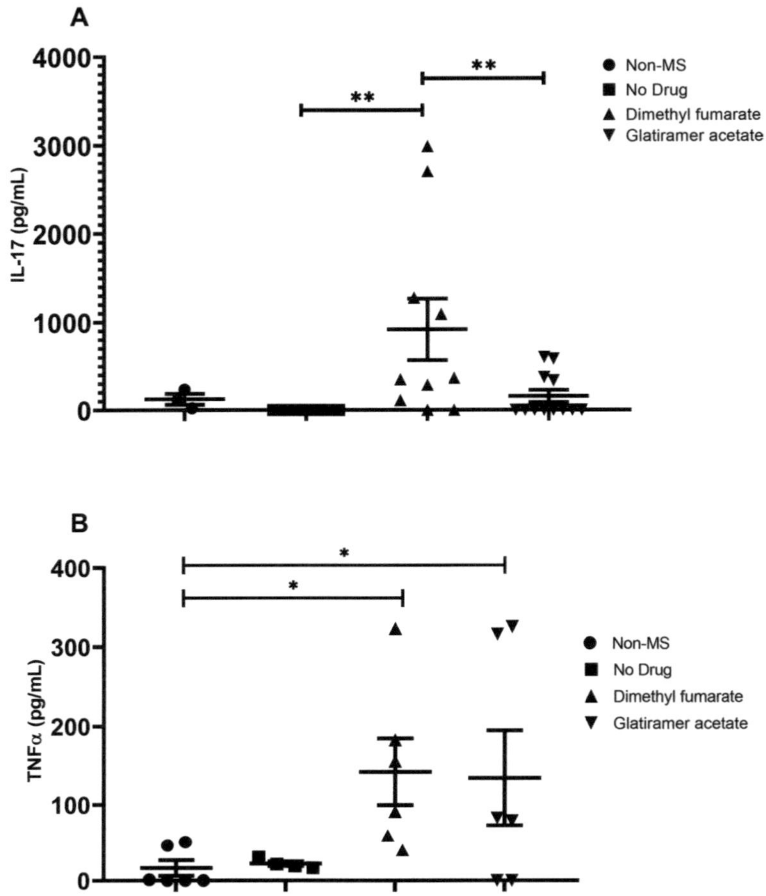

Figure 3.
Scatterplots of serum cytokines IL-17 (A) and TNFα (B) measured by ELISA tests (pg/ml) in RR-multiple sclerosis patients receiving DMTs or no drug; controls include volunteer non-multiple sclerosis subjects. Data was analyzed using one-way ANOVA with subject comparisons made by Newman-Keuls tests. Significantly different at $p < 0.05$ (*) and $p < 0.01$ (**).

in RR-multiple sclerosis, specifically IL-17, IL-17A, and TNFα [67–71]. Inclusion criteria restricted our analyses to RR-MS subjects to those receiving glatiramer acetate or dimethyl fumarate. A few RR-multiple sclerosis subjects in this study were only prescribed LDN as an off-label product.

The restricted access to blood samples and corresponding patient data in this retrospective study limited the findings, as did inclusion of RR-multiple sclerosis patients on no drug. No rationale was reported in the REDCap database to explain why the RR-multiple sclerosis patients had denied therapy. It is conjured that some multiple sclerosis patients who have stabilized over a long period of time request to be removed from therapy.

The focus of this study was to determine the relationship between serum expression levels of endogenous neuropeptides, specifically OGF, and a select group of pro-inflammatory cytokines. OGF levels in the serum of RR-multiple sclerosis subjects declined with age and were not associated with the length of disease. In general, the OGF levels of RR-multiple sclerosis patients using DMTs, or those on no therapy, were substantially lower than RR-multiple sclerosis subjects on LDN. This relationship between OGF and RR-multiple sclerosis has been reported previously [51], suggesting that the biotherapeutic LDN treatment is producing enkephalins. Clinical studies have reported that LDN treatment resulted in perceived increased

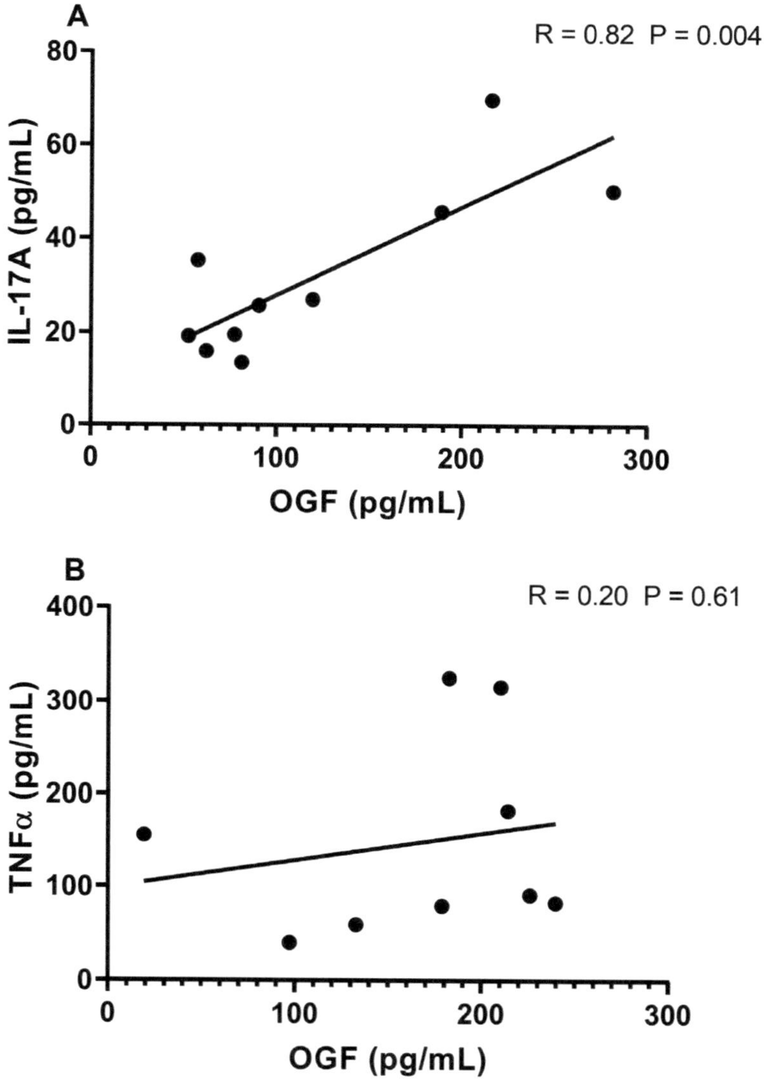

Figure 4.
Associations of cytokine expression between IL-17A (pg/ml) and OGF (pg/ml) (A) or TNFα (pg/ml) and OGF (B) for RR-multiple sclerosis subjects receiving a DMT. Data were analyzed by Pearson's Correlation Coefficient (R) tests. P values less than 0.05 were considered significant.

quality of life [42, 43] and stabilization of disease symptomatology [44]. A second neuropeptide, β-endorphin, is known as the "feel-good" hormone and has been reported to increase during exercise and pregnancy [72] and to increase during multiple sclerosis remission [73]. In this study, β-endorphin levels were comparable in all subjects suggesting that these RR-multiple sclerosis patients had stabilized endorphins. Based on the scatter gram plots of individual expression levels of endorphin, some of the individuals in the glatiramer acetate group may have been in remission. Moreover, whereas OGF levels fluctuate with RR-multiple sclerosis and different therapies, β-endorphin does not appear to be altered by DMTs in RR-multiple sclerosis.

The proinflammatory cytokine IL-17 may be a prime indicator of RR-multiple sclerosis progression [69, 71]. The IL-17 family of cytokines is produced by $CD4^+$ T-helper cells known as Th17 cells. At least 7 polymorphisms have been identified, with IL-17A and IL-17F most frequently associated with neutrophils activation in autoimmunity [67, 69]. IL-17A has been identified in the CNS following migration of Th17 cells in response to a pro-inflammatory event [74]. Clinical studies have reported that IL-17A may be responsible for breakdown of the blood-brain barrier facilitating the entrance of other inflammatory cytokines into the CNS [71]. IL-17A has been shown in preclinical studies to accelerate glial activation leading to neuroinflammation and neurodegeneration [68]. Thus, it would be expected that IL-17A levels may be lowest in RR-multiple sclerosis individuals who are in remission or most responsive to therapy [67]. Moreover, recent preclinical studies have reported that both IL-17A and IL-17F increase pro-inflammatory cytokine IL-6 secretion [70].

In the present study, TNFα, a proinflammatory marker has been shown to increase in RR-multiple sclerosis [75, 76] and to be consistently elevated regardless of the status of disease type (i.e., clinically isolated syndrome, primary progressive, or relapsing-remitting), with serum levels 40–50% higher in multiple sclerosis subjects relative to controls. Preclinical studies have reported an association between TNFα and impaired memory in mice with EAE [77] and implicated astrocyte signaling as the downstream target of overexpression of the cytokine. Despite studies whereby TNFα knockdown mice had more severe EAE [69] and therapeutic administration of the cytokine protected against the disease [74], this cytokine is reported to be a major contributor to cognitive deficits related to late stages of multiple sclerosis. In the present study, age, gender, number of relapses, or length of disease had no effect of TNFα levels, but in general, the expression levels of this cytokine were elevated in RR-multiple sclerosis subjects relative to cohorts of RR-multiple sclerosis patients presumably in remission or non-multiple sclerosis.

LDN is an off-label therapeutic used in substantially lower dosages than prescribed for drug overdose or alcohol use (3 vs. 50 mg). Its use is increasing worldwide [78, 79] and is consistently reported to be well-tolerated over extended periods of time [46]. Small clinical trials have reported few, if any, side effects [42, 43]. In this study, OGF serum levels appear to be correlated with IL-17A. Alternatively, whereas β-endorphin has been associated with the propensity to avoid alcohol or opioids, it was not related to RR-multiple sclerosis. The serum levels of cytokines IL-17A and TNFα did not appear to be discriminating biomarkers at least with the current population of RR-multiple sclerosis subjects. Perhaps with additional study, and possibly other DMTs, these cytokines will be able to discern progression of disease.

3. Conclusions

In summary, the preclinical and clinical data illustrate that enkephalin levels (i.e., OGF) are decreased in animals with EAE and humans with relapsing remitting multiple sclerosis. LDN as a biotherapy is associated with elevating enkephalins and from all aspects, appears to reduce symptomatology of multiple sclerosis. LDN therapy to upregulate the body's own production of enkephalins has been shown by a number of clinical trials to be a safe adjuvant, or primary, treatment for RR-multiple sclerosis. LDN continues to be associated with stabilizing multiple sclerosis and does not appear to interfere with other disease-modifying therapies. Whether enkephalin levels directly or indirectly alter the therapeutic pathways is unclear at this time. Moreover, it is difficult to determine at this point whether specific disease-modifying therapies are more advantageous for manipulating enkephalin levels. However, it is evident that restored serum enkephalin expression is associated with reduced inflammatory cytokines and better patient outcome. Moving forward, studies will be conducted to determine the mechanistic role of

OGF in modulating both pro and anti-inflammatory cytokines. Collectively the data from published studies as well as the new data presented in this report demonstrate that the biotherapeutic LDN and resulting enkephalin (specifically OGF) levels play a role in disease progression of multiple sclerosis. By integrating animal model work and patient serum analysis, future studies will try and understand the role of OGF during initiation of disease and definitive diagnosis of disease. The efficacy of LDN alone needs to be evaluated in prospective, randomized, controlled studies, but unfortunately this design is not forthcoming as most physicians will prescribe the off-label drug based on its safety record.

Acknowledgements

This research was supported in part by a generous gift from The Paul K. and Anna E. Shockley Family Foundation, and private donations to the Penn State LDN Fund.

The authors acknowledge the support of Indira Purushothaman from the McLaughlin and Zagon lab as well as Syndi Reed and Trang Doan from the Institute of Personalized Medicine at Penn State College of Medicine.

Author declaration

At the time of preparation of this manuscript, PJM, ISZ, and CLP had no personal or financial conflicts or disclosures, and GAT was on the speaker bureau for Biogen, but had no equity interest in the product (Tecfidera®).

Author details

Chirag L. Patel, Ian S. Zagon, Gary A. Thomas and Patricia J. McLaughlin*
The Pennsylvania State University College of Medicine, Hershey, Pennsylvania, United States

*Address all correspondence to: pxm9@psu.edu

References

[1] Chen AY, Chonghasawat AO, Leadholm KL. Multiple sclerosis: Frequency, cost, and economic burden in the United States. Journal of Clinical Neuroscience. 2017;**45**:18-186

[2] Leray E, Moreau T, Fromont A, Edan G. Epidemiology of multiple sclerosis. Revue Neurologique (Paris). 2015;**172**:3-13

[3] Belbasis L, Bellou V, Evangelou E, Ioannidis JPA, Tzoulaki I. Environmental risk factors and multiple sclerosis: An umbrella review of systematic reviews and meta-analyses. The Lancet. Neurology. 2015;**14**:263-273

[4] Ascherio A, Munger KL. Epidemiology of multiple sclerosis: From risk factors to prevention—An update. Seminars in Neurology. 2016;**36**(2):103-114

[5] Nourbakhsh B, Mowry EM. Multiple sclerosis risk factors and pathogenesis. CONTINUUM Lifelong Learning in Neurology. 2019;**25**(3):596-610

[6] Jog NR et al. Association of Epstein-Barr virus serological reactivation with transitioning to systemic lupus erythematosus in at-risk individuals. Annals of the Rheumatic Diseases. 2019;**78**(9):1235-1241

[7] Handel AE, Williamson AJ, Disanto G, Dobson R, Giovannoni G, Ramagopalan SV. Smoking and multiple sclerosis: An updated meta-analysis. PLoS One. 2011;**6**(1):1-6

[8] Salzer J, Hallmans G, Nyström M, Stenlund H, Wadell G, Sundström P. Smoking as a risk factor for multiple sclerosis. Multiple Sclerosis Journal. 2013;**19**(8):1022-1027

[9] Riise T, Nortvedt MW, Ascherio A. Smoking is a risk factor for multiple sclerosis. Neurology. 2003;**61**(8):1122-1124

[10] Ramagopalan SV et al. Association of smoking with risk of multiple sclerosis: A population-based study. Journal of Neurology. 2013;**260**:1778-1781

[11] Bashinskaya VV, Kulakova OG, Boyko AN, Favorov AV, Favorova OO. A review of genome-wide association studies for multiple sclerosis: Classical and hypothesis-driven approaches. Human Genetics. 2015;**134**:1143-1162

[12] Sawcer S et al. Genetic risk and a primary role for cell-mediated immune mechanisms in multiple sclerosis. Nature. 2011;**476**(7359):214-219

[13] Hemmer B, Kerschensteiner M, Korn T. Role of the innate and adaptive immune responses in the course of multiple sclerosis. Lancet Neurology. 2015;**14**:406-419

[14] Milo R, Miller A. Revised diagnostic criteria of multiple sclerosis. Autoimmunity Reviews. 2014;**13**:518-524

[15] Hollenbach JA, Oksenberg JR. The immunogenetics of multiple sclerosis: A comprehensive review. Journal of Autoimmunity. 2015;**64**:13-25

[16] Howard J, Trevick S, Younger DS. Epidemiology of multiple sclerosis. Neurologic Clinics. 2016;**34**:919-939

[17] McDonald WI et al. Recommended diagnostic criteria for multiple sclerosis: Guidelines from the international panel on the diagnosis of multiple sclerosis. Annals of Neurology. 2001;**50**(1):121-127

[18] Sand IK. Classification, diagnosis, and differential diagnosis of multiple

sclerosis. Current Opinion in Neurology. 2015;**28**(3):193-205

[19] Polman CH et al. Diagnostic criteria for multiple sclerosis: 2010 revisions to the McDonald criteria. Annals of Neurology. 2011;**69**:292-302

[20] McNicholas N, Hutchinson M, McGuigan C, Chataway J. 2017 McDonald diagnostic criteria: A review of the evidence. Multiple Sclerosis and Related Disorders. 2018;**24**:48-54

[21] Aktas O, Wattjes MP, Stangel M, Hartung HP. Diagnosis of multiple sclerosis: Revision of the McDonald criteria 2017. Nervenarzt. 2018;**89**(12):1344-1354

[22] Brownlee WJ, Hardy TA, Fazekas F, Miller DH. Diagnosis of multiple sclerosis: Progress and challenges. Lancet. 2017;**389**:1336-1346

[23] Arrambide G et al. The value of oligoclonal bands in the multiple sclerosis diagnostic criteria. Brain. 2018;**141**(4):1075-1084

[24] Makhani N et al. Oligoclonal bands increase the specificity of MRI criteria to predict multiple sclerosis in children with radiologically isolated syndrome. Multiple Sclerosis Journal—Experimental, Translational and Clinical. 2019;**5**(1):2055217319836664

[25] Weinshenker BG. Natural history of multiple sclerosis. Annals of Neurology. 1994;**36**(Suppl 1):S6-S11

[26] Richards RG, Sampson FC, Beard SM, Tappenden P. A review of the natural history and epidemiology of multiple sclerosis: Implications for resource allocation and health economic models. Health Technology Assessment. 2002;**6**(10):1-45

[27] Gelfand JM. Multiple sclerosis: Diagnosis, differential diagnosis, and clinical presentation. Handbook of Clinical Neurology. 2014;**122**(2014):269-290

[28] Okuda DT et al. Radiologically isolated syndrome: 5-year risk for an initial clinical event. PLoS One. 2014;**9**(3):1-9

[29] Dendrou CA, Fugger L, Friese MA. Immunopathology of multiple sclerosis. Nature Reviews. Immunology. 2015;**15**:545-558

[30] Baecher-Allan C, Kaskow BJ, Weiner HL. Multiple sclerosis: Mechanisms and immunotherapy. Neuron. 2018;**97**(4):742-768

[31] Malpass K. Multiple sclerosis: 'Outside-in' demyelination in MS. Nature Reviews Neurology. 2012;**8**(2):61

[32] Lucchinetti CF et al. Inflammatory cortical demyelination in early multiple sclerosis. The New England Journal of Medicine. 2011;**365**(23):2188-2197

[33] Sospedra M, Martin R. Immunology of multiple sclerosis. Seminars in Neurology. 2016;**36**(2):115-127

[34] Vasileiadis GK et al. Regulatory B and T lymphocytes in multiple sclerosis: Friends or foes? Autoimmunity Highlights. 2018;**9**(9):1-15

[35] Hartung HP, Aktas O, Menge T, Kieseier BC. Immune regulation of multiple sclerosis. Handbook of Clinical Neurology. 2014;**122**(2014):3-14

[36] Garg N, Smith TW. An update on immunopathogenesis, diagnosis, and treatment of multiple sclerosis. Brain and Behavior: A Cognitive Neuroscience Perspective. 2015;**5**(9):1-13

[37] Steinman L. Immunology of relapse and remission in multiple sclerosis. Annual Review of Immunology. 2014;**32**:257-281

[38] Pierrot-Deseilligny C, Souberbielle J-C. Vitamin D and multiple sclerosis: An update. Multiple sclerosis and related disorders. 2017;**14**:35-45

[39] Gholamzad M et al. A comprehensive review on the treatment approaches of multiple sclerosis: Currently and in the future. Inflammation Research. 2019;**68**:25-38

[40] Ciotti JR, Cross AH. Disease-modifying treatment in progressive multiple sclerosis. Current Treatment Options in Neurology. 1940;**20**:12

[41] Brown N, Panksepp J. Low-dose naltrexone for disease prevention and quality of life. Medical Hypotheses. 2009;**72**:333-337

[42] Cree BAC, Kornyeyeva E, Goodin DS. Pilot trial of low-dose naltrexone and quality of life in multiple sclerosis. Annals of Neurology. 2010;**68**(2):145-150

[43] Sharafaddinzadeh N, Moghtaderi A, Kashipazha D, Majdinasab N, Shalbafan B. The effect of low-dose naltrexone on quality of life of patients with multiple sclerosis: A randomized placebo-control trial. Multiple Sclerosis. 2010;**16**(8):964-969

[44] Ludwig MD, Turel AP, Zagon IS, McLaughlin PJ. Long-term treatment with low dose naltrexone maintains stable health in patients with multiple sclerosis. Multiple Sclerosis Journal—Experimental, Translational and Clinical. 2016;**2**:1-11

[45] Gironi M et al. A pilot trial of low-dose naltrexone in primary progressive multiple sclerosis. Multiple Sclerosis. 2008;**14**:1076-1083

[46] Turel AP, Oh KH, Zagon IS, McLaughlin PJ. Low dose naltrexone for treatment of multiple sclerosis: A retrospective chart review of safety and tolerability. Journal of Clinical Psychopharmacology. 2015;**35**(5):609-611

[47] Li Z, You Y, Griffin N, Feng J, Shan F. Low-dose naltrexone (LDN): A promising treatment in immune-related diseases and cancer therapy. International Immunopharmacology. 2018;**61**:178-184

[48] Toljan K, Vrooman B. Low-dose naltrexone (LDN)-review of therapeutic utilization. Medical Science. 2018;**6**:82

[49] McLaughlin PJ, Zagon IS. Duration of opioid receptor blockade determines biotherapeutic response. Biochemical Pharmacology. 2015;**97**:236-246

[50] Donahue RN, McLaughlin PJ, Zagon IS. Low-dose naltrexone targets the opioid growth factor-opioid growth factor receptor pathway to inhibit cell proliferation: Mechanistic evidence from a tissue culture model. Experimental Biology and Medicine. 2011;**236**:1036-1050

[51] Ludwig MD, Zagon IS, McLaughlin PJ. Serum [Met5]-enkephalin levels are reduced in multiple sclerosis and restored by low-dose naltrexone. Experimental Biology and Medicine. 2017;**242**:1-10

[52] Ludwig MD, Zagon IS, McLaughlin PJ. Modulation of the OGF-OGFr pathway alters cytokine profiles in experimental autoimmune encephalomyelitis and multiple sclerosis. Experimental Biology and Medicine. 2018;**243**:361-369

[53] Campbell AM, Zagon IS, Mclaughlin PJ. Opioid growth factor arrests the progression of clinical disease and spinal cord pathology in established experimental autoimmune encephalomyelitis. Brain Research. 2012;**1472**:138-148

[54] Hammer LA, Zagon IS, McLaughlin PJ. Treatment of a relapse-remitting model of multiple sclerosis with opioid growth factor. Brain Research Bulletin. 2013;**98**:122-131

[55] Hammer LA, Zagon IS, McLaughlin PJ. Improved clinical behavior of established relapsing-remitting experimental autoimmune encephalomyelitis following treatment with endogenous opioids: Implications for the treatment of multiple sclerosis. Brain Research Bulletin. 2015;**112**:42-51

[56] Hammer LA, Waldner H, Zagon IS, McLaughlin PJ. Opioid growth factor and low-dose naltrexone impair central nervous system infiltration by CD4+ T lymphocytes in established experimental autoimmune encephalomyelitis a model of multiple sclerosis. Experimental Biology and Medicine. 2016;**241**:71-78

[57] Zagon IS, Rahn KA, Turel AP, McLaughlin PJ. Endogenous opioids regulate expression of experimental autoimmune encephalomyelitis: A new paradigm for the treatment of multiple sclerosis. Experimental Biology and Medicine. 2009;**234**(11):1383-1392

[58] Bruno K et al. Targeting toll-like receptor-4 (TLR4)-an emerging therapeutic target for persistent pain states. Pain. 2018;**159**(10):1908-1915

[59] Li J, Csakai A, Jin J, Zhang F, Yin H. Therapeutic developments targeting toll-like receptor-4-mediated neuroinflammation. ChemMedChem. 2016;**11**(2):154-165

[60] Patten DK, Schultz BG, Berlau DJ. The safety and efficacy of low-dose naltrexone in the management of chronic pain and inflammation in multiple sclerosis, fibromyalgia, Crohn's disease, and other chronic pain disorders. Pharmacotherapy: The Journal of Human Pharmacology and Drug Therapy. 2018;**38**(3):382-389

[61] Smith JP et al. Treatment of advanced pancreatic cancer with opioid growth factor: Phase I. Anti-Cancer Drugs. 2004;**15**(3):203-209

[62] Smith JP, Field D, Bingaman SI, Evans R, Mauger DT. Safety and tolerability of low-dose naltrexone therapy in children with moderate to severe Crohn's disease: A pilot study. Journal of Clinical Gastroenterology. 2013;**47**(4):339-345

[63] Smith JP et al. Therapy with the opioid antagonist naltrexone promotes mucosal healing in active Crohn's disease: A randomized placebo-controlled trial. Digestive Diseases and Sciences;**56**(7):2088-2097

[64] Younger J, Noor N, McCue R, MacKey S. Low-dose naltrexone for the treatment of fibromyalgia: Findings of a small, randomized, double-blind, placebo-controlled, counterbalanced, crossover trial assessing daily pain levels. Arthritis and Rheumatism. 2013;**65**(2):529-538

[65] Guest PC, Rahmoune H. Blood bio-sampling procedures for multiplex biomarkers studies. Methods in Molecular Biology. 2017;**1546**:161-168

[66] Tuck MK et al. Standard operating procedures for serum and plasma collection: Early detection research network consensus statement standard operating procedure integration working group. Journal of Proteome Research. 2009;**8**(1):113-117

[67] Bălaşa R, Bajko Z, Huţanu A. Serum levels of IL-17A in patients with relapsing-remitting multiple sclerosis treated with interferon-β. Multiple Sclerosis Journal. 2013;**19**(7):885-890

[68] Bartlett HS, Million RP. Targeting the IL-17-TH17 pathway. Nature

Reviews. Drug Discovery. 2014; **14**(1):11-12

[69] Wang X et al. The properties of cytokines in multiple sclerosis: Pros and cons. The American Journal of the Medical Sciences. 2018;**356**:552-560

[70] Noack M, Beringer A, Miossec P. Additive or synergistic interactions between IL-17A or IL-17F and TNF or IL-1β depend on the cell type. Frontiers in Immunology. 2019;**10**:1726

[71] Setiadi AF et al. IL-17A is associated with the breakdown of the blood-brain barrier in relapsing-remitting multiple sclerosis. Journal of Neuroimmunology. 2019;**332**:147-154

[72] Csontos K, Rust M, Höllt V, Mahr W, Kromer W, Teschemacher HJ. Elevated plasma β-endorphin levels in pregnant women and their neonates. Life Sciences. 1979;**25**(10):835-844

[73] Gironi M et al. β endorphin concentrations in PBMC of patients with different clinical phenotypes of multiple sclerosis. Journal of Neurology, Neurosurgery, and Psychiatry. 2003;**74**(4):495-497

[74] Liu J et al. TNF is a potent anti-inflammatory cytokine in autoimmune-mediated demyelination. Nature Medicine. 1998;**4**(1):78-83

[75] Mokhtarzade M, Ranjbar R, Majdinasab N, Patel D, Molanouri Shamsi M. Effect of aerobic interval training on serum IL-10, TNFα, and adipokines levels in women with multiple sclerosis: Possible relations with fatigue and quality of life. Endocrine. 2017;**57**(2):262-271

[76] Mulero P et al. Netrin-1 and multiple sclerosis: A new biomarker for neuroinflammation? European Journal of Neurology. 2017;**24**(9):1108-1115

[77] Habbas S et al. Neuroinflammatory TNFa impairs memory via astrocyte signaling in brief pathological levels of TNFa trigger signaling in astrocytes, leading to synaptic alterations and memory deficits in a mouse model of multiple sclerosis. Article neuroinflammatory TNFa impairs memory via astrocyte signaling. Cell. 2015;**163**

[78] Raknes G, Småbrekke L. A sudden and unprecedented increase in low dose naltrexone (LDN) prescribing in Norway. Patient and prescriber characteristics, and dispense patterns. A drug utilization cohort study. Pharmacoepidemiology and Drug Safety. 2017;**26**(2):136-142

[79] Zagon IS, McLaughlin PJ. Multiple sclerosis: Perspectives in treatment and pathogenesis. Brisbane (AU): Codon Publications; 2017

Chapter 7

Traditional Chinese Medicine in Geriatrics, Evidences, and the Guideline

Koh Iwasaski

Abstract

The average life span of Japanese is 90 years. So that Japan is an unprecedented super-aging society. However, healthy life span is 10 years shorter than life span. Many spend an average of 10 years in frailty. People become frail, and reached to "geriatric syndrome."

Keywords: traditional chinese medicine, elderly, dementia, aspiration pneumonia, constipation

1. Geriatric syndrome

Geriatric syndromes include many symptoms caused by aging, such as dementia, depression, delirium, incontinence, vertigo, falls, spontaneous bone fractures, failure to thrive, and neglect and abuse. Geriatric syndromes are associated with reduced life expectancy. To be considered a geriatric syndrome, these conditions must interfere with a person's daily life.

In ancient China, people considered this phenomenon as Qi (気) deficiency in Kidney organ (shen xu, 腎虚). Qi is energy and signaling using energy. Kidney in traditional Chinese medicine (TCM) is very different from Kidney in Western medicine. TCM kidney is somewhat base of life. Human inherits essence of life (jing, 精) from his/her parents and keeps it all his/her life. When jing runs out, people die. TCM kidney is the box keeping jing. When people become old, the jing in TCM kidney decreases, and the function of whole body goes down. This is the reason of aging and geriatric syndrome. These thoughts were written in the famous ancient medical text book Huan di nei jing (黄帝内経), written in BC 2nd ~ 1st century. That is to say, TCM had geriatric medicine in 2000 years ago. How can we keep jing in TCM kidney? People seeked the ways, from unexpected to some herbal drugs, training methods.

Here, we introduce some evidences of TCM for geriatric syndrome and clinical practice guideline from Japan Geriatrics Society. How can we treat geriatric syndrome using traditional Chinese Medicine?

2. Dementia

In China, dementia is called as chidai (痴呆). Zhang Jing yue (張景岳) developed this term in his text book Jing yue guan Su (景岳全書), in12th century. But Zhang Jing yue considered chidai as acquired symptoms. He thought that unstable emotion induced chidai. In Qing (清) era, 19th century, Wang Qing Ren (王清任)

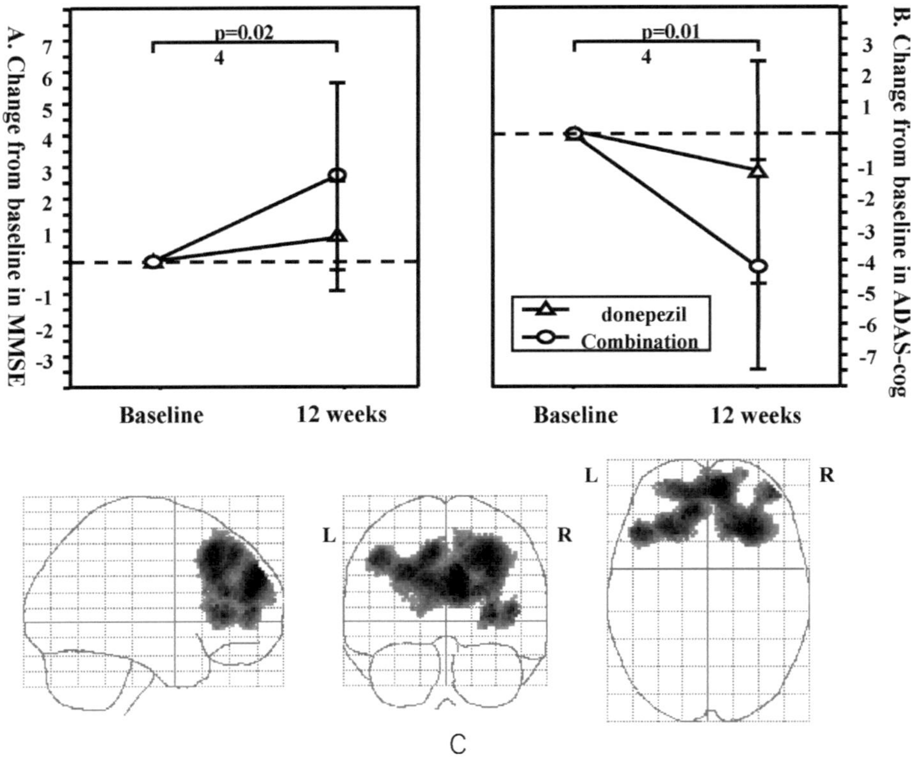

Figure 1.
Change of MMSE(lt) and ADAScog of 2 groups, donepezil plus KUT combination (○) vs. donepezil only (△). Combination group showed significant improvement to single donepezil group. Colored areas in the brain reveal areas in which significant blood flow increases in the combination group.

considered that chidai was caused by brain atrophy. Wang Qing Ren is the first man who described dementia in a scientific manner.

We demonstrated that a combinatorial use of donepezil plus Jia wei weng dan tang (加味温胆湯), was more beneficial than donepezil alone in both cognition and brain perfusion (**Figure 1**) in demented people. Although cholinergic-related adverse effects might be expected, such events did not occur in the combination group. Therefore, despite a small sample size and a short observation period study, donepezil and Jia wei weng dan tang may work synergistically in a safe fashion to enhance an availability of acetylcholine [1].

Same time, we showed that bawei dihuan wang (八味地黄丸、BDW) could improve the cognitive function of Alzheimer disease patient. **Figure 2** shows that BDW improves Mini Mental Score Examination about 2.5 in the treatment period [2]. BDW was described in the ancient text book Jin kui Yao lue (金匱要略) written by Zhan Zhong jing (張仲景) in 2nd century. He wrote that this recipe delayed aging, i.e., effective for Qi (気) deficiency in Kidney organ (shen xu, 腎虚). Therefore, it is used for geriatric syndrome and frailty of aged people. It contains Rehmaniae Radix, Corni Fructus, Dioscoreae Rhizoma, Alismatis Rhizoma, Hoelen, Moutan Cortes, Cinnamomi Cortes and Aconi tuber.

3. Traditional Chinese medicine for behavioral and psychological symptoms of dementia (BPSD)

Behavioral and psychological symptoms of dementia (BPSD) is the serious clinical problem of dementia. Usually major tranquilizers are used, but they

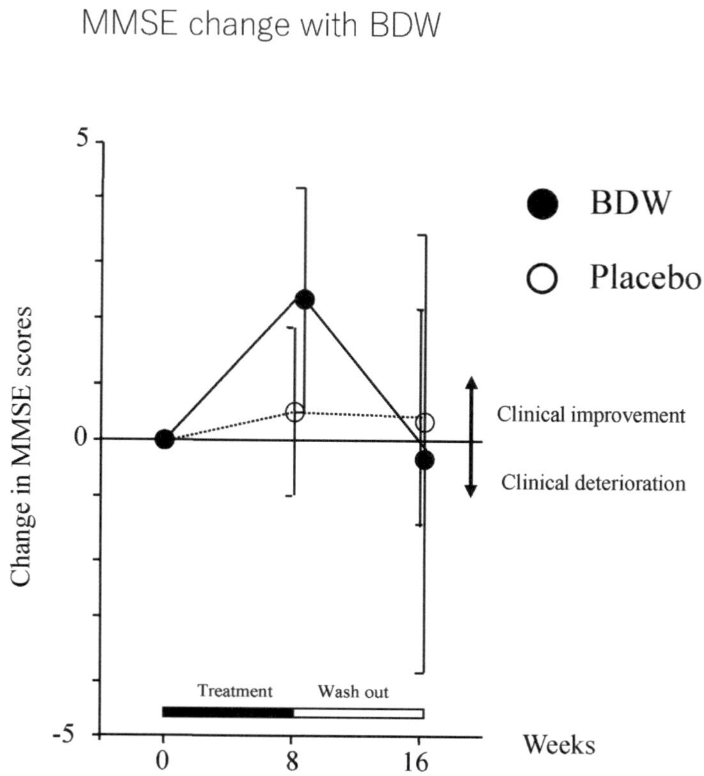

Figure 2.
Changes of MMSE of BDW and placebo groups. BDW improves mini mental score examination about 2.5 in the treatment period.

cause extrapyramidal side effects. We reported that Yigan San (抑肝散) could improve BPSD without extrapyramidal side effects [3]. Mild-to-severe demented patients who had BPSD (18 men and 34 women; age 80.3 ± 9.0 [mean ± SD] years) were investigated. Participants were randomly assigned to the YGS group (n = 27) or control (drug-free) group (n = 25) and treated for 4 weeks. The Neuropsychiatric Inventory (NPI) test for the assessment of BPSD. Meanwhile, cognitive function was estimated by the Mini-Mental State Examination (MMSE), and ADL by the Barthel Index were tested at baseline and the end of the treatment. The frequency of extrapyramidal symptoms (EPS) and other adverse events were recorded. All participants in both groups completed the trial. In the control group, 11 patients required treatment with tiapride hydrochloride because of deterioration of BPSD.

Significant improvements BPSD (from 37.9 ± 16.1 to 19.5 ± 15.6, mean ± SD) (**Figure 3**) and Barthel index (from 56.4 ± 34.2 to 62.9 ± 35.2) were observed in the YGS group, but not in the control group. MMSE was not changed in both groups. EPS were not observed in either group, but dizziness and impaired postural sway were observed in 6 patients treated in control group, may be caused by tiapride hydrochloride. At the same time, we also found that Yigan San could improve typical hallucination in Dementia with Lewy Bodies (DLB), as shown in **Figure 4** [4].

Yigan San was developed by Xue Ji (薛己) in 16th century. He devised this recipe for emotional liability of children. But this recipe was not widely spread in China, and Japanese doctors in Edo era applied it to adults. They found that it is effective for persons who are easy to anger. I applied it to some demented patients who easily anger. Therefore, I carried out Randomized Control Trial (RCT) described above. Now then, we found 219 papers with key word "yokukansan (Japanese

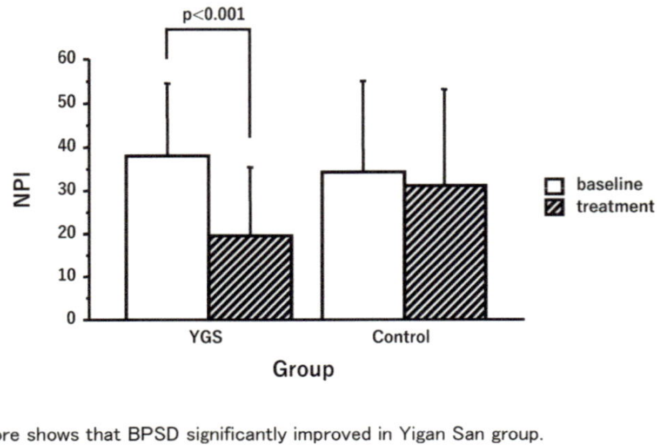

Figure 3.
Changes of NPI in the YGS group and control. NPI significantly improved from baseline to endpoint only in the YGS group.

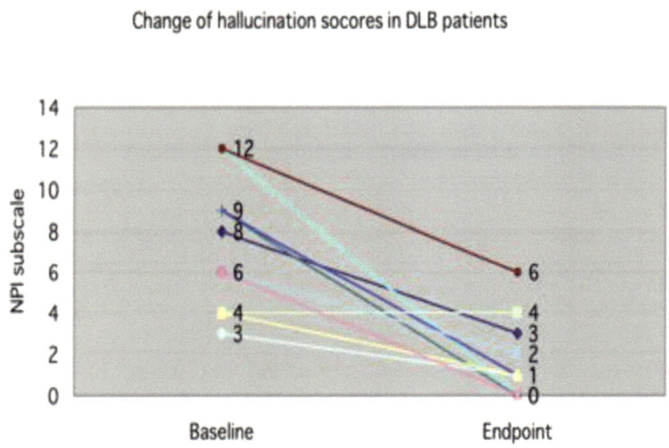

Figure 4.
Change of hallucination sub score of NPI in DLB patients. Hallucination improved by YGS treatment.

name of Yigan San)." Nakatani Y et al. reported that Yigan San has a neuroprotective effect [5]. Yigan San contains Atractylodis Lanceae Rhizama, Hoelen, Cnidii Rhizoma, Angelicae Radix, Bupleuri Radix, Glycyrrhizae Radix, and Uncariae Ramulus et Uncus. Active ingredients are not sure but Ikarashi Y et al. reported that Geissoschizine methyl ether (GM) in Uncaria hook and 18β-glycyrrhetinic acid (GA) in Glycyrrhiza may concern to several pharmacological actions of YiGan San [6].

4. Aspiration pneumonia

Pneumonia is now the 4th reason of death of Japanese, and most of them are aspiration pneumonia in the elderly. Absence or attenuation of the cough [7] and swallowing [8] reflex in elderly patients causes micro aspiration. We investigated the effects of Banxia Houpu Tang (半夏厚朴湯、BHT), on the swallowing [9] (**Figure 5**) and cough [10] (**Figure 6**) reflexes in elderly stroke patients. Finally, we found that BHT reduced pneumonia risk in the elderly [11]. Elderly participants

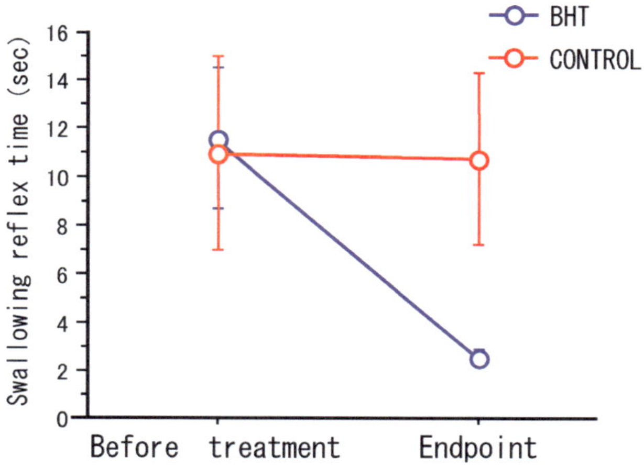

Figure 5.
Changes of the swallowing reflex in BHT and the control groups. The reflex significantly improved the time (shortened) only in the BHT group.

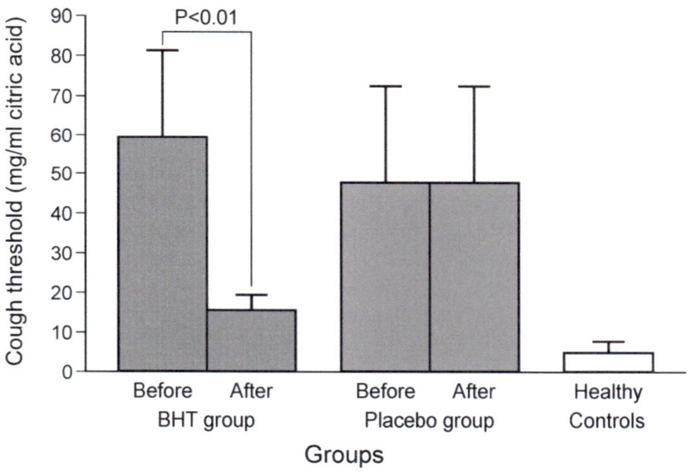

Figure 6.
Change of the cough reflex in BHT treated and the control groups. The threshold of the reflex significantly shortened (improved) in the BHT group.

who had history of aspiration pneumonia (mean age 84.0, M:F = 28:67) were randomly assigned to the BHT treatment group (n = 47) or the control group (n = 48) and took BHT or placebo for 12 months. The occurrence of pneumonia, mortality due to pneumonia, and the daily amount of self-feeding were measured. As a result, four participants in the BHT group developed pneumonia, and one of them died as a result, while 14 participants in the control group developed pneumonia, and 6 of them died. There was a significant difference between the two groups in pneumonia onset ((**Figure 7**, *P* = .008), and a tendency toward significance in pneumonia-related mortality (*P* = .05). The relative risk of pneumonia in the BHT group compared with the control group was 0.51 (95% confidence interval (CI 0.27–0.84, *P* = .008) and that of death from pneumonia was 0.41 (95% CI = 0.10–1.03, *P* = .06). No adverse events were observed from treatment with BHT. The BHT group was able to maintain self-feeding better than the control group (*P* = .006). Very recently, the suppressing effect of BHT for aspiration pneumonia was confirmed by double blind RCT [12].

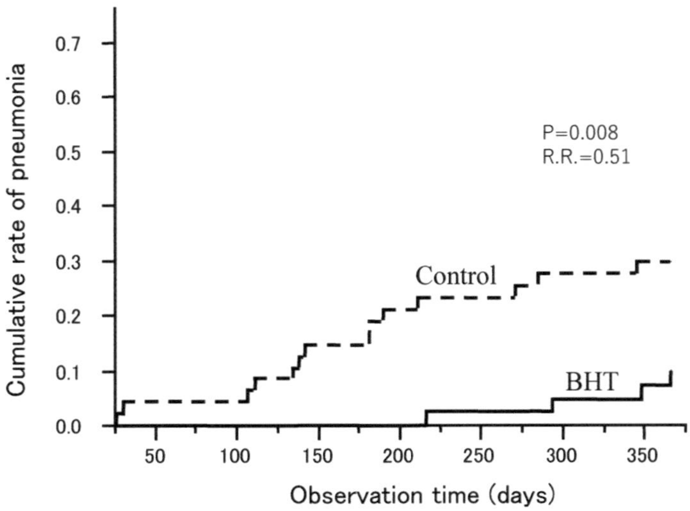

Figure 7.
Cumulative rate of pneumonia in BHT treatment group and the control group. There is a significant difference in pneumonia occurrence rate between the groups.

BHT was described in Jin kui Yao lue (金匱要略) by Zhan Zhong jing (張仲景) in 2nd century. It contains Pinelliae Tuber, Hoelen, Magnoliae Cortex, Perillae Herba, and Zingiberis Rhizoma. It is written that when women feel something block her throat, try this recipe. Now it is considered as throat dysesthesia, and BHT is widely applied to neurosis, depression, and psychophysiological disorder.

5. Chronic constipation

There were over 1.34 million patients suffering from cerebrovascular diseases in 2008 reported by Ministry of Health, Labour and Welfare in Japan. Poststroke patients often cause constipation. Stratified by stroke severity on the National Institutes of Health Stroke Scale, the incidence of constipation in poststroke patients were reported from 38.9% to 88.2% [13]. Poststroke patients with functional constipation, assessed by the Rome III criteria were recruited in a study on the effects of the traditional Chinese medicine Da Jian Zhong Tang (大建中湯) on constipation. Thirty-four patients (17 men and 17 women; mean age: 78.1 ± 11.6 years) were randomly assigned to 2 groups; all patients received conventional therapy for constipation, and patients in the Da Jian Zhong Tang group received 15 g/day of Da Jian Zhong Tang for 4 weeks. We recorded Constipation Scoring System (CSS) points and the Gas Volume Score (GVS) (the measure of the intestinal gas volume calculated from plain abdominal radiographs) before and after a 4-week observation period. The total score on the CSS improved significantly in the Da Jian Zhong Tang group compared to the control ($p < 0.01$) (**Figure 8**). In addition, some CSS subcategories (defecation frequency, feeling of incomplete evacuation, and need for enema/disimpaction) significantly improved in the Da Jian Zhong Tang group ($p < 0.01$, $p = 0.049$, and $p = 0.03$, respectively). The GVS was also significantly reduced in the Da Jian Zhong Tang group (**Figure 9**, $p = 0.03$) [14]. Da Jian Zhong Tang was also described in Jin kui Yao lue (金匱要略) by Zhan Zhong jing (張仲景) in 2nd century. Zhan Zhong jing wrote that this recipe was effective for patients who felt severe abdominal pain, abdominal coldness and gut sharply moved. It is very

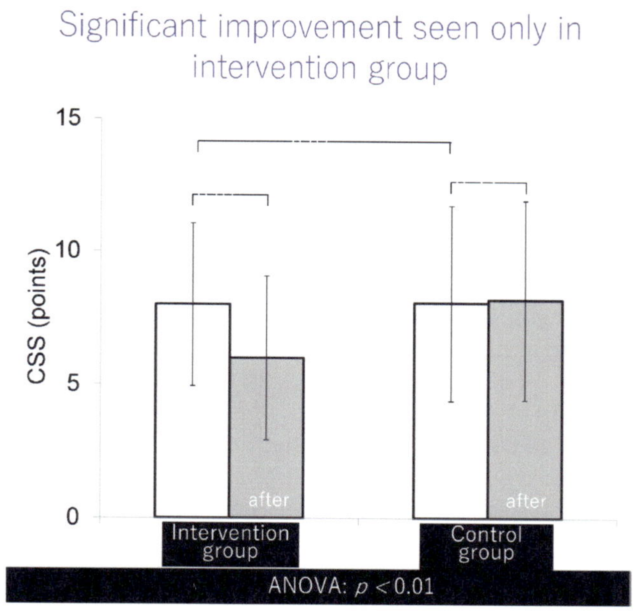

Figure 8.
Change of CCS points in the Da Jian Zhong tang treated group and the control. CSS significantly reduced (improved) in Da Jian Zhong tang group.

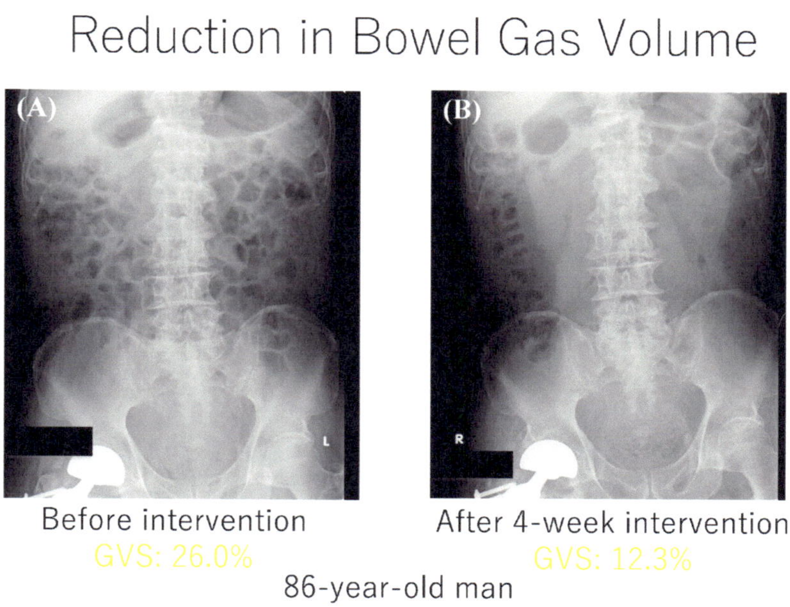

Figure 9.
Bowel gas volume at baseline and the endpoint of Da Jian Zhong tang treatment (a case).

alike to ileus, and this recipe had been used for ileus prevention after abdominal surgery. Da Jian Zhong Tang contains Ginseng Radix, Zanthoxyli Fructus, and Zingiberis Siccatum Rhizoma.

6. Guideline

Concerning these evidences, Japan Geriatric Society treated traditional medicine as the independent chapter in their guideline 2015 [15]. As a result, Yigan San,

Banxia houpu Tang, Da Jian Zhong Tang, Buzhongyiqi Tang (補中益気湯), and Ma Zi Ren Wan (麻子仁丸) covering by Japanese national insurance, were reviewed and found to have a high Quality of evidence for the elderly (**Table 1**). In these 5 recipes, I already explained Yigan San, Banxia houpu Tang, Da Jian Zhong Tang above. Buzhongyiqi Tang was developed by Li Dong yuan (李東垣) in 13th century. He promoted the theory that disease results from the inhibition of digestive functions. In his book Pi wei lun (脾胃論), he wrote as below. Mongolian army attacked his country and closed in the capital many months. At that time, severe infectious disease spread in the capital and many people died. Doctors could not treat the disease. Then he thought that people went down because of food deficiency. Their digestion deteriorated and immune function declined so that infectious disease did not recover. Then he developed Buzhongyiqi Tang and treated many patients. Buzhongyiqi Tang was assessed in two small, open labeled RCTs [16, 17], the findings of which suggested that it improved systemic inflammation and nutritional status in elderly patients with chronic obstructive pulmonary disease and reduced systemic inflammation. It represents a unique therapeutic strategy to improve nutritional status and control chronic inflammation, something lacking in Western medicine. Buzhongyiqi Tang contains Astragali radix, Atractylodis Lanceae Rhizoma, Ginseng Radix, Angelicae radix, Bupleuri Radix, Cimicifugae Rhizoma, and Zingiberis Rhizoma.

Ma Zi Ren Wan (麻子仁丸) is purgative, very easy to use for the elderly. It was described in 2 books, Jin kui Yao lue and Shang ha lun (傷寒論), both written by Zhang Zhong jin. It contains Rhei Rhizoma, Aurantii Fructus Immaturus, Armeniacae Semen, Magnoliae Cortes, Paeoniae Radix, and Cannabidis Semen. The effect as purgative was proved the double blinded RCT [18].

Medicines	Ingredients	Effects	Attention	QoE and RS
Yigan San (Chinese), Yokukansan (Japanese), (抑肝散)	蒼朮: Atractylodis Lanceae 当帰: Angelicae Radix 茯苓: Hoelen 柴胡: Bupleuri Radix 川芎: Cnidii Rhizoma 甘草: Glycyrrhizae Radix 釣藤鈎: Uncariae Uncis Cum Ramulus	Yigan San improves the BPSD of dementia patients (AD, VD and DLB), and is particularly effective for DLB-related hallucinations.	Hypokalemia could occur in 6 % of cases.	QoE: moderate RS: strong
Banxia houpu Tang (Chinese), Hangekobokuto (Japanese), (半夏厚朴湯)	半夏: Pinelliae Tuber 蘇葉: Perillae Herba 茯苓: Hoelen 生姜: Zingiberis Rhizoma 厚朴: Magnoliae Cortex	Banxia houpu tang (BHT) reduced the aspiration pneumonia risk in elderly patients with dementia and maintained self-feeding.	None	QoE: moderate RS: strong
Dajianzhong Tang (Chinese), daikenchuto (Japanese), (大建中湯)	乾姜: Zingiberis Siccatum Rhizoma 山椒: Zanthoxyli Fructus 人参: Panacis Ginseng Radix 膠飴: Maltose	Dajianzhong Tang is effective for defecation control in post-stroke patients.	Interstitial pneumonia, and, rarely, liver dysfunction.	QoE: moderate RS: strong
Buzhongyiqi Tang (Chinese), hochuekkito (Japanese), (補中益気湯)	黄耆: Astragali Radix 大棗: Zizyphi Fructus 蒼朮: Atractylodis Lanceae 陳皮: Aurantii Nobilis Pericarpium 人参: Panacis Ginseng Radix 甘草: Glycyrrhizae Radix 当帰: Angelicae Radix 升麻: Cimicifugae Rhizoma 柴胡: Bupleuri Radix 生姜: Zingiberis Rhizoma	Buzhongyiqi Tang improved systemic inflammation and nutritional status in patients with COPD	It contains licorice and may cause hypokalemia	QoE: low RS: weak
Ma Zi Ren Wan, (Chinese), mashiningan (Japanese), Hemp seed pill (HSP) (English) (麻子仁丸)	麻子仁: Cannabis Fructus 杏仁: Armeniacae Semen 大黄: Rhei Rhizoma 厚朴: Magnoliae Cortex 枳実: Aurantii Fructus Immaturus 芍薬: Paeoniae Radix	HSP is safe and effective for alleviating functional constipation. According to the study in reference 31, those in the HSP group benefited in terms of increased complete spontaneous bowel movement, relief in the severity of constipation and straining, and an effective reduction in the use of rescue therapy when compared with placebo. HSP is safe and effective for alleviating functional constipation.	HSP is a very safe purgative. No adverse events were reported.	QoE: moderate RS: strong

Table 1.
Screening tool to alert doctors to right treatment (START).

7. Conclusion

As mentioned above, evidences of traditional medicine for geriatrics accumulated little by little, and a part of it is accepted modern medical doctors. Systematic education for traditional medicine and medical care needed.

Author details

Koh Iwasaski
Natorikumanodoh Hospital, Japan

*Address all correspondence to: iwasaki.koh67@gmail.com

References

[1] Maruyama M, Tomita N, Iwasaki K, Ootsuki M, Matsui T, Nemoto M, Okamura N, Higuchi M, Tsutsui M, Suzuki T, Seki T, Kaneta T, Furukawa K, Arai H. Benefits of combining donepezil plus traditional Japanese herbal medicine on cognition and brain perfusion in Alzheimer's disease: a 12-week observer-blind, donepezil monotherapy controlled trial. J Am Geriatr Soc. 2006 May;54(5):869-71.

[2] Iwasaki K, Kobayashi S, Chimura Y, Taguchi M, Inoue K, Cho S, Akiba T, Arai H, Cyong JC, Sasaki H. A randomized, double-blind, placebo-controlled clinical trial of the Chinese herbal medicine "ba wei di huang wan" in the treatment of dementia. J Am Geriatr Soc. 2004 Sep;52(9):1518-21.

[3] Iwasaki K, Satoh-Nakagawa T, Maruyama M, Monma Y, Nemoto M, Tomita N, Tanji H, Fujiwara H, Seki T, Fujii M, Arai H, Sasaki H. A randomized, observer-blind, controlled trial of the traditional Chinese medicine Yi-Gan San for improvement of behavioral and psychological symptoms and activities of daily living in dementia patients. J Clin Psychiatry. 2005 Feb;66(2):248-52

[4] Iwasaki K, Maruyama M, Tomita N, Nemoto M, Fujiwara H, Seki T, Fujii M, Kodama M, Arai H Effects of the Traditional Chinese Herbal Medicine for Cholinesterase inhibitor-Resistant Visual Hallucinations and Neuropsychiatric Symptoms in patients with Dementia with Lewy Bodies. J of Clin Psychiatry 66:12, Dec 2005. 1612-13

[5] Nakatani Y, Amano T, Yamamoto H, Sakai N, Tsuji M, Takeda H. Yokukansan enhances the proliferation of B65 neuroblastoma. J tradit Complement Med 2016 Feb 22;7(1) 34-44

[6] Ikarashi Y, Mizoguchi K. Neuropharmacological efficacy of the traditional Japanese Kampo medicine yokukansan and its active ingredients. Pharmacol Therapy 2016 Oct;166:84-95.

[7] Sekizawa K, Ujiie Y, Itabashi S. Sasaki H, Takishima T. Lack of cough reflex in aspiration pneumonia. Lancet 1990; 335:1228-1229.

[8] Nakagawa H, Sekizawa K, Ujiie Y, Sasaki H, Takishima T. Risk of aspiration pneumonia in the elderly. Chest 1993; 103:1636-1637.

[9] Iwasaki K, Wang Q, Nakagawa T, Suzuki T, Sasaki H. The Traditional Chinese Medicine Banxia Houpo Tang improves swallowing reflex. Phytomedicine 1999; 6(2):103-106

[10] Iwasaki K, Cyong JC, Kitada S, Kitamura H, Ozeki J, Satoh Y, Suzuki T, Sasaki H. A traditional Chinese herbal medicine, banxia houpo tang, improves cough reflex of patients with aspiration pneumonia. J Am Geriatr Soc. 2002 Oct;50(10):1751-2.

[11] Iwasaki K, Kato S, Monma Y,, Niu K,, Ohrui T, Okitsu R, Higuchi S, Ozaki S , Kaneko N, Seki T, Nakayama K, Furukawa K, Fujii M, Arai H. A Pilot Study of Banxia Houpu Tang, a Traditional Chinese Medicine, for Reducing Pneumonia Risk in Older Adults with Dementia J Am Geriatr Soc. 2007 Dec;55(12):2035-40

[12] Kawago K, Nishibe T, Shindo S, Inoue H, Motohashi S, Akasaka J, Ogino H. A Double-Blind Randomized Controlled Trial to Determine the Preventive Effect of Hangekobokuto on Aspiration Pneumonia in Patients Undergoing Cardiovascular Surgery. Ann Thorac Cardiovasc Surg 2019;25:318-325. doi: 10.5761/atcs.oa.19-00128 [published Online First: Epub Date].

[13] Y. Su, X. Zhang, J. Zeng, Pei Z, Cheung R, Zhou Q, Ling L, Yu J, Tan J, Zhang Z. "New-onset constipation at acute stage after first stroke: incidence, risk factors, and impact on the stroke outcome," *Stroke, vol.* 40, no. 4, pp. 1304-1309, 2009.

[14] Numata T, Takayama S, Tobita M, Ishida S, Katayose D, Shinkawa M, Oikawa T, Aonuma T, Kaneko S, Tanaka J, Kanemura S, Iwasaki K, Ishii T, Yaegashi N. Traditional Japanese medicine daikenchuto improves functional constipation in poststroke patients. Evid Based Complement Alternat Med. 2014

[15] Takayama S, Iwasaki K. Systematic review of traditional Chinese medicine for geriatrics. Geriatr Gerontol Int. 2017 May;17(5):679-688.

[16] Shinozuka N, Tatsumi K, Nakamura A, Terada J, Kuriyama T. The traditional herbal medicine Hochuekkito improves systemic inflammation in patients with chronic obstructive pulmonary disease. J Am Geriatr Soc 2007;55:313-314.

[17] Tatsumi K, Shinozuka N, Nakayama K, Sekiya N, Kuriyama T, Fukuchi Y. Hochuekkito improves systemic inflammation and nutritional status in elderly patients with chronic obstructive pulmonary disease. J Am Geriatr Soc 2009;57:169-170.

[18] Cheng CW, Bian ZX, Zhu LX, Wu JC, Sung JJ. Efficacy of a Chinese herbal proprietary medicine (Hemp Seed Pill) for functional constipation. Am J Gastroenterol 2011;106:120-129.